Strategic Approaches to HIV/AIDS Prevention and Control

Strategic Approaches to HIV/AIDS Prevention and Control

V. Ramamurthy

AUTHORSPRESS

Worldwide Circulation through Authorspress Global Network
First Published 2004
by Authorspress

E-35/103, Jawahar Park
Laxmi Nagar, Delhi-110 092

e-mail: authorspress@yahoo.com

Typeset in NewCenturySchlbk by Chitra Computers

Strategic Approaches to HIV/AIDS Prevention and Control
ISBN 81-7273-185-X

Printed in India at Tarun Offset, Delhi.

Preface

Twenty years after the first clinical evidence of acquired immuno-deficiency syndrome was reported, AIDS has become the most devastating disease humankind has ever faced. Since the epidemic began, more than 60 million people have been infected with the virus. Today HIV is prevalent in all parts of the world and has spread from urban to rural areas, and from individuals practising high risk behaviours to the general population. Even though science and technology have enabled us to achieve tremendous progress in all spheres of life, it cannot find out a vaccine to protect the community from this dreadful virus, till today.

The sense of common purpose in the worldwide struggle against HIV/AIDS has intensified in the past few years. The political momentum to tackle AIDS has grown. Public opinion in many countries has been mobilised by the media, non-governmental organisations, activists, doctors, economists, and people living with HIV/AIDS. Communities and nations are progressively taking the lead in responding to the epidemic with increased political commitment, resources and institutional initiatives.

Prevention of HIV/AIDS is one of the most important objective of almost all nations. Health education and behaviour modification is the prime focus of action for interrupting transmission. It is therefore important to have information and education programmes for all men and women, including adolescents and children, especially aimed at those who are at greater risk of HIV infection. It is also important to have facilities for detection and treatment of other sexually transmitted infections and to encourage an environment that promotes free and frank dissemination of information without stigmatisation and discrimination against suspected/known cases of HIV/AIDS.

Comprehensive HIV/AIDS programmes should be planned, which address prevention as well as access to care, treatment and support, and thus serve as effective mechanisms in halting the spread of the HIV/AIDS epidemic. An understanding and supportive environment that improves the quality of life of people living with HIV/AIDS is a hallmark of these comprehensive programmes.

The prevention efforts must be buttressed by well-supported community responses that include people living with HIV/AIDS, religious groups, and traditional and trusted leaders. In the context of more effective HIV treatment and the drop in anti-retroviral drug prices, prevention must be linked to the provision of care and support. As the epidemic is constantly shifting, prevention efforts must be tailored to developments in the epidemic, on the research front, and to evaluations that confirm success or failure.

The book shares positive ideas and creative solutions for action to stop the spread of HIV/AIDS. In addition to discussing methods and strategies of HIV/AIDS prevention, it covers a wide range of public health, psycho-social, ethical, and public policy concerns related to HIV and AIDS. Professionals working to prevent HIV and AIDS including local service providers, NGOs and family care givers will find this book useful in their efforts to provide effective and innovative care and support to people living with HIV/AIDS. The information contained in this work will also help to correct the myths and biases readers' may have internalised regarding the epidemic.

Editor

Contents

1

HIV/AIDS: Global Trends

According to the recent estimates of UNAIDS, around the world an estimated 40 million people are living with HIV/AIDS, 2.5 million of them children. Over the next decade, without effective treatment and care, they will join the ranks of the more than 20 million people who have died of AIDS since the first clinical evidence of HIV/AIDS was reported in 1981. It is equally clear that the vast majority of people (including those living in countries with high national HIV prevalence) have not yet acquired the virus. Enabling them to protect themselves against HIV, and providing adequate and affordable treatment and care to people living with the virus, represent two of the biggest challenges facing humankind today.

Table 1

Global summary of the HIV/AIDS epidemic (December 2003)

Number of people living with HIV/AIDS	
Total	40 million (34 – 46 million)
Adults	37 million (31 – 43 million)
Children under 15 years	2.5 million (2.1 – 2.9 million)
People newly infected with HIV in 2003	
Total	5 million (4.2 – 5.8 million)
Adults	4.2 million (3.6 – 4.8 million)
Children under 15 years	700.000 (590 000 – 810.000)
AIDS deaths in 2003	
Total	3 million (2.5 – 3.5 million)
Adults	2.5 million (2.1 – 2.9 million)
Children under 15 years	500,000 (420 000 – 580.000)

REGIONAL TRENDS

HIV/AIDS marks a severe development crisis in almost all countries of the world, especially in sub-Saharan Africa, which remains by far the worst-affected region in the world. Beyond sub-Saharan Africa, the epidemics of HIV/AIDS continue to grow in China, Indonesia, Papua New Guinea, Vietnam, several Central Asian Republics, the Baltic States, and North Africa. Vietnam, for example, provides fresh evidence of how an HIV/AIDS epidemic can erupt suddenly wherever significant levels of injecting drug use occurs. It has joined a growing list of countries in Asia, Eastern Europe, the Middle East and Latin America, where injecting drug use has primed HIV/AIDS epidemics. In such settings, as in the epidemic generally, stigma and discrimination rank high among the obstacles that hinder efforts to turn the tide of AIDS.

Sub-Saharan Africa

Sub-Saharan Africa remains by far the region worst-affected by the HIV/AIDS epidemic. In 2003, an estimated 26.6 million people in this region were living with HIV, including the 3.2 million who became infected during the past year. AIDS killed approximately 2.3 million people in 2003. Unlike women in other regions in the world, African women are considerably more likely—at least 1.2 times—to be infected with HIV than men. Among young people aged 15–24, this ratio is the highest: women were found to be two-and-a-half times as likely to be HIV-infected as their male counterparts, according to six recent national surveys. These discrepancies have been attributed to several factors. They include the biological fact that HIV generally is more easily transmitted from men to women (than vice versa). As well, sexual activity tends to start earlier for women, and young women tend to have sex with much older partners.

HIV prevalence varies considerably across the continent—ranging from less than 1 per cent in Mauritania to almost 40 per cent in Botswana and Swaziland. More than one in five pregnant women are HIV-infected in most countries in Southern Africa, while elsewhere in sub-Saharan Africa median HIV prevalence in antenatal clinics exceeded 10 per cent in a few countries. And while sustained prevention efforts in a few countries in West and East Africa continue to demonstrate that HIV/AIDS can be checked with human intervention, signs that similar inroads might be building in Southern Africa remain tenuous, at best.

Eastern Europe and Central Asia

The AIDS epidemic in Eastern Europe and Central Asia shows no signs of abating. Some 230,000 people were infected with HIV in 2003, bringing the total number of people living with the virus to 1.5 million. AIDS claimed an estimated 30,000 lives in the past year. The worst-affected are the Russian Federation, Ukraine, and the Baltic States (Estonia, Latvia and Lithuania), but HIV continues to spread in Belarus, Moldova and Kazakhstan, while more recent epidemics are now evident in Kyrgyzstan and Uzbekistan. HIV prevalence continues to rise in the Russian Federation, which remains saddled with the worst epidemic in this region. By the end of 2002, a cumulative total of 229,000 people had been diagnosed with HIV. Almost a quarter of that total was added in 2002 alone, indicating that the epidemic is growing at a fearsome rate. Moreover, these reported cases almost certainly grossly underestimate the number of people living with HIV.

Asia and the Pacific

Over 1 million people in Asia and the Pacific acquired HIV in 2003, bringing to an estimated 7.4 million the number of people now living with the virus. A further 500,000 people are estimated to have died of AIDS in 2003. National adult HIV prevalence is still under 1 per cent in the majority of this region's countries. Several countries in the region are so large and populous that national aggregations can obscure serious epidemics in some provinces and states.

Table 2. Regional HIV/AIDS Statistics and Features, 2003

Region	*Adults and children living with HIV/AIDS*	*Adults and children newly infected with HIV*	*Adult prevalence (%)**	*Adult & child deaths due to AIDS*
Sub-Saharan Africa	25.0 – 28.2 million	3.0 – 3.4 million	7.5 – 8.5	2.2 – 2.4 million
North Africa & Middle East	470,000 – 730,000	43,000 – 67,000	0.2 – 0.4	35,000 – 50,000
South & South-East Asia	4.6 – 8.2 million	610,000 – 1.1 million	0.4 – 0.8	330,000 – 590,000
East Asia & Pacific	700,000 – 1.3 million	150,000 – 270,000	0.1 – 0.1	32,000 – 58,000
Latin America	1.3 – 1.9 million	120,000 – 180,000	0.5 – 0.7	49,000 – 70,000
Caribbeans	350,000 – 590,000	45,000 – 80,000	1.9 – 3.1	30,000 – 50,000
Eastern Europe & Central Asia	1.2 – 1.8 million	180,000 – 280,000	0.5 – 0.9	23,000 – 37,000
Western Europe	520,000 – 680,000	30,000 – 40,000	0.3 – 0.32	600 – 3,400
North America	790,000 – 1.2 million	36,000 – 54,000	0.5 – 0.7	12,000 – 18,000
Australia & New Zealand	12,000 – 18,000	700 – 1,000	0.1 – 0.1	<100
TOTAL	40 million (34 – 46 million)	5 million (4.2 – 5.8 million)	1.1% (0.9 – 1.3%)	3 million (2.5 – 3.5 million)

* The proportion of adults (15 to 49 years of age) living with HIV/AIDS in 2003, using 2003 population numbers.

Source: UNAIDS, 2003

The HIV/AIDS picture in South Asia remains dominated by the epidemic in India, where between 3.82 and 4.58 million people were infected nationally by the end of 2002. In neighbouring Bangladesh and Nepal, national HIV prevalence has remained under 1 per cent, but risky behaviour in parts of the population is so extensive that it could be just a matter of time before wider epidemics erupt. In the Nepalese capital, Kathmandu, HIV epidemics are centred around injecting drug users and sex workers, most of them young. Among the former, HIV prevalence of up to 68 per cent has been detected in recent years, while, among the latter, prevalence is around 17 per cent.

Latin America and the Caribbeans

More than 2 million people are now living with HIV in Latin America and the Caribbeans, including the estimated 200,000 that contracted HIV in the past year. At least 100,000 people died of AIDS in the same period—the highest regional death toll after sub-Saharan Africa and Asia. HIV/AIDS is well entrenched in this region, with national HIV prevalence at least 1 per cent in 12 countries, all of them in the Caribbean Basin. The most recent national estimates showed HIV prevalence among pregnant women reaching or exceeding 2 per cent in six of them: the Bahamas, Belize, the Dominican Republic, Guyana, Haiti, and Trinidad and Tobago. In contrast, most of the other countries of the region have highly concentrated epidemics, notably in South America where Brazil is home to the vast majority of people living with HIV in the region.

Two of the region's most serious epidemics are on Hispaniola Island—in Haiti and the Dominican Republic. Stricken with the lowest health and other development indicators in the entire region, Haitians' woes are being aggravated dramatically by the AIDS epidemic, which is claiming an estimated 30,000 lives a year and has left some 200,000 children orphaned by AIDS. Haiti's national HIV prevalence levels have remained at 5–6 per cent since the late 1980s. The factors contributing to this apparent levelling off of national HIV prevalence are unclear, although it must be noted that sentinel surveillance has shown that HIV prevalence levels vary dramatically. With about 60 per cent of the population under 24 years of age, much scope exists for renewed growth in Haiti's mainly hetero-sexually transmitted epidemic. Condom use is very low among young people, despite evidence that HIV/AIDS knowledge is comparatively strong.

Middle East and North Africa

The notion that this region has sidestepped the global HIV epidemic is not borne out by the latest estimates, which indicate that 55,000 people acquired HIV infection in the past year, bringing to 600,000 the total number of people living with HIV/AIDS in the Middle East and North Africa. AIDS killed a further 45,000 people in 2003. There is the potential for a considerable rise in the number of HIV infections in this region. By far the most seriously affected country at present is the Sudan—specifically the south, where a mainly heterosexual epidemic is well under way. Available data indicate a national adult HIV prevalence of more than 2 per cent, but conflict is hampering both surveillance of the epidemic and the mounting of a potentially effective response. The last round of surveillance data showed that HIV prevalence among pregnant women was six to eight times higher in the south of Sudan, compared to Khartoum.

In most other countries, HIV spread in this region appears to be nascent, although scant surveillance data in several countries could mean that serious outbreaks in certain populations may be being missed. There also appears to be significant movement of HIV-infected persons between some countries. More than half of those officially reported to have HIV in Tunisia, for example, are believed to have crossed the border from Libya to seek anti-retroviral treatment and/or to undergo drug rehabilitation.

The epidemic threatens to expand along diverse routes in the region, including through blood transfusions and blood collection. Universal precautions and blood screening have greatly reduced the risks of transmission in health-care settings in most countries, but HIV transmission through blood and blood products remains a potentially significant danger in some. Also of concern is the rise in HIV infections among injecting drug users, particularly in Bahrain, Libya and Iran, while HIV infections linked to this mode of transmission have been reported in Algeria, Egypt, Kuwait, Morocco, Oman and Tunisia.

High-income Countries

The total number of people living with HIV continues to rise in high-income countries, largely due to widespread access to anti-retroviral treatment. It is estimated that 1.6 million people are living with HIV in these countries—a figure that includes the 80,000 who were newly infected in 2003. AIDS claimed approximately 18,000 lives in the past year. The number of annual AIDS deaths has continued to slow in high-income countries, including those in Western Europe, due to the widespread availability of anti-retroviral treatment. There is mounting evidence that prevention activities in several high-income countries are not keeping pace with the changes occurring in the spread of HIV. Such shortcomings are most evident where HIV is lodged also among marginalised sections of populations, including immigrants and refugees.

In the United States of America, around half of the approximately 40,000 new infections annually are occurring among African-Americans (12 per cent of the country's population), with African-American women accounting for an increasing proportion of new infections. Many of the women do not engage in high-risk behaviour, but are contracting HIV through unsafe sex with their male partners—a significant share of whom also have sex with men or inject drugs. Analysing data from 11 States, a recent US Centers for Disease Control and Prevention study found that 34 per cent of HIV-positive African-American men said they had sex with both women and men. However, only a small proportion of HIV positive African-American women reported knowing that their partners also had sex with men. The secrecy surrounding such overlapping risk behaviour seems rooted mainly in the stigma that remains attached to homosexuality. The costs are steep: AIDS is now the leading cause of death for African-American women aged 25–34. According to the Centres for Disease Control, some 90 per cent of young urban HIV-positive African-American men who have sex with other men are unaware of their seropositive status. Overall, it is estimated that fully one-quarter of the 850,000–950,000 people living with HIV/AIDS in the USA are unaware that they are HIV-positive.

Sex between men remains an important aspect of the epidemic in most high-income countries. In Germany, Greece and the Netherlands, it is the most common mode of HIV transmission, while in the United States of America and in Australia it accounted for 42 per cent and 86 per cent of new HIV diagnoses, respectively. Yet, the resurgence of other sexually transmitted infections in Australia, Japan, Western Europe and the United States of America points to a revival of high-risk sexual behaviour—especially among young people, including men who have sex with men. The prevention programmes that had achieved notable success in limiting HIV transmission in the 1990s, especially among men who have sex with men, appear to have been shifted to the back burner in many high-income countries.

ESTIMATING POPULATIONS AT RISK FOR HIV

The difficulty in focusing prevention efforts appropriately is especially pronounced in countries where HIV remains largely concentrated among sub-populations whose behaviour puts them at high risk for contracting and transmitting HIV. Many governments find it politically difficult to invest in services for injecting drug users, men who have sex men and female sex workers and the clients they serve. And yet in most countries in the world, these sub-populations remain among the most important focal points for effective HIV prevention.

In Asia, Latin America and Eastern Europe, where HIV is more heavily concentrated in sub-populations with defined risk behaviours, more and more governments are now investing in surveillance systems that track the distribution of the virus and the behaviours that spread it in the hardest-hit populations. However even the best existing surveillance systems have one central weakness. While they can measure the level of risk behaviour, HIV and STI infection in a given sub-population, they cannot give any indication of the absolute size of the sub-population itself.

Many countries have begun to attempt to estimate the size of populations at high risk for HIV. No standardised methodologies are currently available to guide this process, and many different approaches have been tried. In an effort to synthesize the "state of the art" for population size estimation in one region where HIV is concentrated predominantly in groups with high risk behaviours, the Joint United Nations Programme on HIV/AIDS (UNAIDS) and the United States Agency for International Development (USAID) sponsored a workshop on estimation methods in Asia.

Many countries are in the process of building up robust surveillance systems, tracking the spread of HIV and of other sexually transmitted infections (STIs), as well as of the sexual and injecting behaviours that carry a risk of transmitting HIV. While much remains to be done in strengthening surveillance, many countries are now able to estimate prevalence of HIV and risk behaviours in certain groups with some confidence.

However, only few countries have any reliable idea how many people inject drugs in the country. That means it isn't possible to estimate either how many people are already infected through injecting (and so how many injectors may be in need of HIV-related care services), or how many more may be at risk unless effective prevention is introduced. Broadly, reasons for developing reliable estimates of the size of populations at high risk for HIV can be grouped into two major areas: policy and programming.

The area of policy encompasses advocacy, response planning and resource allocation, plus estimations of numbers infected with HIV and projections of the burden of disease. The area of programming encompasses intervention planning, measurement of coverage, and monitoring and evaluation of interventions. Different methods may be appropriate for different goals. For policy purposes, national estimates are frequently needed, where as local estimates will often do the job if the goal is to design or monitor specific prevention or care programmes.

The very first use of population size estimation may be to alert policymakers to the existence and the magnitude of a sub-population that may be at risk for HIV. Local governments rarely act on national-level information. They are driven, rather, by local votes and local concerns. If it can be demonstrated that significant sub-populations at risk for HIV exist in their own region, action is more likely to follow.

In some large countries, size estimation exercises are taking place at the local level with no central coordination, limiting the ability to arrive at robust national estimates. As this area of surveillance develops, the central surveillance authority may want to make recommendations for standard definitions and methods so that local estimates can more easily be used effectively at a national level.

Once the extent of the potential problem has been made explicit through sound estimates of the number of people potentially affected, it is far easier to argue persuasively for funding for prevention and care interventions. If both male and female sex workers have the same average numbers of clients each, then it probably makes sense to dedicate more resources to prevention efforts in commercial sex between men and women than between men and men. Population size information is therefore an important ingredient in deciding how resources should be allocated between groups. Perhaps the most politically sensitive of the uses of estimates of the size of at-risk populations is in determining the number of people infected with HIV in a country.

In many parts of Asia, and in some parts of Latin America and Eastern Europe, proportion of major sub-populations are infected with HIV. Important populations are sometimes ignored completely or severely understated when calculating how many people in a country are living with HIV. On the other side of the coin, lack of reliable estimates leaves the door open for wild guesses and hyperbole from organisations interested in maximising the resources allocated to populations with which they work.

Many organisations maintain global databases on HIV, drug use and other related risks. And many countries have undertaken to report information regularly to these organisations for inclusion in their databases. While meeting global reporting requirements should never be the driving force for any kind of data collection, there is a principle of "enlightened self-interest" at stake. If countries submit estimates of HIV infection that are based on sound surveillance systems and well-documented, credible estimates of the size of various at-risk populations, these estimates will be included in the databases and made available globally to donors and others who may be considering allocating resources in the field of HIV. This may increase international contributions to a national response, and avoid international institutions coming up with their own estimates, independently of national procedures.

HIV epidemics are not static, in part because the behaviours that drive them are subject to change. Some of this change may be in response to HIV prevention programmes, some may not. Some countries have, for example, recorded a recent rapid rise in the proportion of drug users reporting the use of non-injected amphetamine type substances. If this rise means drug users are switching from injectible to non-injectible drugs, the implications may be a reduced emphasis on IDUs as a key population for HIV prevention and care. If, however, the number of IDUs is constant and the rising proportion of drug users not injecting reflects not a switch but a rise in the overall number of people taking drugs, then the policy implications are different.

Some countries have to know the relative size of different at-risk populations so that they can plan their overall response and allocate resources efficiently. But knowing the size of specific populations at a local level is also key to good programme planning, implementation and management.

In recent years, more resources have become available to help prevent HIV and more is known about what works in helping people to reduce particularly risky behaviours. Those changes, combined with a growing realisation that impact on the epidemic as a whole depends on changing the behaviours of a high proportion of those most at risk, have led to a shift away from "pilot projects" and "boutique interventions" and towards prevention programming on a larger scale.

Cheaper, more user-friendly treatments have also increased the demand for widespread provision of care to those affected. More and more, the talk is of "scaling up" and of "achieving coverage". And of course, reaching coverage targets depends on knowing how many people are in need of services.

In many developing countries, a significant proportion of the funding for HIV-related programmes comes from foreign donors or lenders. Many of them have, together with developing country governments, signed up to international targets for HIV prevention, care and service provision such as those associated with the United Nations Special Session on AIDS (UNGASS) declaration of 2001. And they expect to be able to measure progress towards those targets.

There are several excellent reasons for increasing efforts to estimate the size of populations at risk for HIV. But they come with a caveat. Population size estimation alone does not solve the problems of HIV planning and programming. Estimates of the size of at-risk populations are meant to be used in conjunction with other sources of information. Many of the purposes given above, especially those surrounding advocacy and resource allocation, can only be fulfilled by combining population estimates with information on HIV prevalence and risk behaviour generated by the surveillance system.

The uses of population size estimation associated with measuring coverage depend on good record-keeping for service delivery. And that in turn depends on there being services in place. In short, the caveat is this: there is little point investing resources in repeatedly estimating the size of at-risk populations unless there is a commitment to provide services for those populations.

HIV and behavioural surveillance systems and at-risk population estimates are likely to be controlled by public health authorities who assume that the information will lead to better HIV prevention and care policies. Other authorities may have different viewpoints. There is a very real possibility that reliable estimates of the numbers of drug injectors, street-based sex workers, gay men etc., will lead not to a public health response but to a law-enforcement response.

The likelihood of this happening of course depends on the national situation, but it should be carefully considered when undertaking—and above all when publicising the results of—population size estimation efforts. A final caveat is that population size estimation methods are designed only to arrive at estimated counts of groups at high risk for HIV. Many methods are based on mathematical calculations, and require no contact with individuals. These methods are certainly not designed to identify individuals who may be members of groups at high risk for HIV, or to facilitate access to those groups for programming.

Issues and Challenges

There are some overall issues which need to be considered in planning population size estimation. These are common to all groups, and to all methodologies. The first and often most difficult issue is in defining the population whose size one wishes to estimate. In public health terms concerned with people whose behaviour puts them at risk for HIV. That may well not be all members of a defined population: there may be significant sub-populations within that group at no risk at all, and in no need of services.

In some countries, physicians and health care workers are among the ranks of injecting drug users. Since they have easy access to sterile injecting equipment and a strong professional motivation to conceal their drug use, they are neither at high risk for HIV infection nor likely to come into contact with any of the locations or data sources that may be used for size estimation. This means they will be excluded from most estimates of drug injecting populations, but since they are not at high risk for HIV, this is not a major concern for HIV programme planners. From an HIV prevention point of view, it would not be worth making a special effort to capture this sub-population.

In other cases, however, it will be important to make estimates separately for different sub-populations within a group that shares a common risk behaviour for HIV, because the various sub-populations may require different HIV prevention and care services. For example, unprotected anal sex between males carries a high risk of HIV transmission, regardless of whether these males identify themselves as transsexuals, transvestites (or even as women), as gay men, or as heterosexual men simply wanting a sexual "change of scene".

Clearly, however, HIV prevention services will have to differ between these groups if they are to be effective. If population size estimations are being undertaken for programme planning and evaluation purposes, they may have to be carried out separately for the different sub-populations involved. Many behaviours that carry a high risk for HIV are very situation-specific. Different cities may have very different patterns of drug use, with heroin injection being the norm in one city while inhalation dominates in another city.

The ethnic majority in the central plains of a country may have a tradition of male sex workers attending temple festivals, while no such tradition exists among the ethnic minorities concentrated in the northern hills. This means it is rarely possible to generalise estimates from one city or region to the rest of the country. National estimation efforts may have to stratify between areas of high, medium and low prevalence of risk behaviours, or may have to aggregate separate estimates from key provinces. Aggregation is not always as easy as it sounds.

One factor that throws off estimates based on the sum of separate regional estimates is migration. Since local level estimates are usually more connected with programme planning and evaluation than with policy, they tend to focus on the total number of people needing services over a given planning cycle, such as a year. If people only sell sex in a city for six months on average before moving to another city where they are considered "new stock" and command higher prices, the annual total will be twice as high as the total at any one time.

More complicated still are sex workers who follow the market on a weekly basis, working in the capital on weekdays but flying to resort islands to serve holidaying clients from neighbouring countries at weekends. Behaviours that carry a risk for HIV are, like all behaviours, subject to change over time. Fashion, the economy, changes in drug routes or tourism patterns, seasonal migration, politics—all can affect the prevalence of risk behaviours and, therefore, the size of the population.

Populations at high risk for HIV are often referred to as "hidden populations" or "hard-to-reach populations", with mixed justification. Brothel based sex workers, for example, are neither hidden nor hard to reach. Middle class drug injectors are usually both. Regular government social service or health workers can conduct enumerations of brothel-based sex workers. That would be almost impossible in the case of drug injectors, where non-government organisations that provide services to the populations have a much better chance of securing some access. In both cases, methods that require contact with the population (such as enumeration, nomination and multiplication methods using multipliers derived from surveys) will benefit from including members of the population itself in the contact team.

Populations at risk for HIV are often in contact with institutions which can provide access either to individuals or to records. Such institutions vary by the population at risk, but may include health and treatment services for drug abuse or STIs, other medical services such as emergency wards, the criminal justice system (including courts and prisons), and broader public institutions such as schools.

The problem with individuals contacted through most institutional settings is that they rarely represent all members of a population at risk. For example, drug treatment programmes typically attract chronic, long term users at the conclusion of their drug using careers. Jails and criminal justice settings also underrepresent newer users, drug users who are not physically dependent and those not involved in criminal activities to support their drug use.

Emergency room samples overrepresent users of more toxic substances. STI services will tend to over represent sex workers with the riskiest behaviour, especially if treatment, rather than routine screening, predominates. Methadone treatment programmes will only yield information about opioid users, private programmes will only include drug users that can afford to be in treatment, and jail records will reflect those drug users engaged in criminal activities and not able to bribe their way out.

Many techniques do, in fact, require some kind of identification of individuals, and identifying individuals at high risk for HIV is often synonymous with identifying individuals engaged in illegal activities. While this information may be safe in the hands of public health officials, it may not be safe in the hands of other groups. The desire to know how many people are at risk for HIV should never be allowed to take precedence over the rights and welfare of the members of the populations at risk.

The danger of a backlash exists not only at the individual but also at the population level, through the mere publication of information about the existence and size of a sub-population.

Even anonymous estimation methods that do not identify individuals in any way can lead to a "spotlight" effect, where the population at risk for HIV is suddenly publicly identified as the 'source' of infection or potential infection. Some countries have moved beyond the stage of targeting sub-populations in a negative way just because of a potential association with HIV, but this is by no means universally true.

NGOs can be fiercely competitive, and many have an interest in seeing estimates of the size of the populations they are serving kept high. In some countries, NGOs have sought to discredit independent surveillance organisations publishing the results of population size estimation exercises based on transparent and robust methods.

Methods of Estimation

There are different methods that can be used, either alone or in combination, to arrive at estimates of the size of populations at high risk for HIV. Each method is described together with its strengths and weaknesses. Census and enumeration methods boil down, in essence, to counting people.

Census methods try to count every individual in a population, for example by visiting every brothel in the country and collecting information on the number of individual sex workers based in each brothel. This has to take place in a very short space of time, since otherwise migration between sites may lead to double counting.

Enumeration methods are very similar, but instead of counting every individual they generally start with a sample frame or list, choose a sample of "units" from within that list, and count only the individuals within those chosen units. The number counted is then scaled up according to the size and structure of the sample frame. In other words they may count the number of brothels, visit a third of them to get an average number of workers per brothel, and then multiply the average number of workers per brothel by the total number of brothels counted.

Census and enumeration methods are mathematically straightforward. Where a good sample frame already exists and where the population of interest is well-defined and visible, census methods can actually be less time-consuming than other, more sophisticated methods, and can give better results. They are especially well-suited to counts at the local level. Census methods are not well suited to hidden populations, or to areas that are geographically diverse and where populations at risk are scattered.

In these situations, it is rarely possible to field a sufficiently large staff to do the count over just a day or two. Enumeration methods share the advantages and disadvantages of census methods, although because they tend to cover a smaller fraction of the population they usually require fewer people. Working with reliable community guides covering relatively small areas, enumeration methods can also reach more "hidden" populations than census methods. In other words, census methods work well when it is possible and feasible to reach everybody in a given sub-population, while enumeration methods work better when it is only possible or feasible to reach a fraction of them.

The most common form of general population survey is the household survey, where a questionnaire is administered to residents of a sample of households drawn from a sample frame that is representative at the national or regional level. In industrialised countries these surveys are sometimes conducted by telephone, but in developing countries they usually involve face-to-face interviews with members of a survey team. Household surveys commonly explore health and nutrition issues, including contraception.

Many countries in Africa and the industrialised world and a few in Asia and Latin America have conducted household surveys of sexual risk behaviour, and a few, mostly in industrialised countries, conduct regular household surveys of drug use. These surveys give a prevalence of risk behaviour among the respondents sampled. Since the sample is known to be representative of a larger population, that prevalence can then be applied to the whole population to give an estimate of the total number of individuals engaging in the behaviour.

Other types of population surveys include surveys of sub-populations at high risk for HIV transmission, most commonly male, female and transsexual sex workers, groups of men likely to be their clients, injecting drug users, and men who have sex with men. Generally, the places where members of a given sub-population gather are mapped, and a random sample of the population of interest at those locations is invited to participate in a survey. The Asian region leads the world in repeated cross-sectional surveys of risk behaviour for HIV, and many other countries also have well-established behavioural surveillance systems in these groups.

Unlike general population surveys, behavioural surveillance in high risk groups cannot, by itself, give an estimation of population size. Whereas general population surveys provide the prevalence of a behaviour among a larger population, the respondents for behavioural surveillance are chosen because they engage in that behaviour (e.g., they are injecting drug users) or because they are more likely than members of the general population to engage in a risk behaviour.

In general, it is easy to construct a sample frame for a general population survey, and easy to calculate exactly how representative the sample is of the general population. This means that results can easily be extrapolated to the entire area covered by a survey—often nationally. Since the methodologies are well established, the results of a general population survey are usually quite easy to defend. General population surveys are, in other words, very robust ways of measuring the prevalence of behaviours which are widespread in the general population.

Arriving at a population size estimate is as simple as applying the prevalence measured in the survey to the population represented in the survey. However most behaviours which carry a high risk for HIV in concentrated HIV epidemics are not very widespread in the general population. Indeed it is the rarity of these behaviours that allows HIV to remain concentrated, rather than to spread widely through the general population. Due to this, the usefulness of household surveys is somewhat limited.

Firstly, household surveys do not include every single household, they select respondents from a sample of households. Where a behaviour is rare, it may not get picked up in a sample survey, unless the sample is very large, because the small number of individuals who practise the behaviour may not be included as respondents, even where selection is random.

Secondly, many of the people engaging in behaviours which carry a high risk for HIV transmission are not in households at all. Sex workers may live in brothels, their clients may be in barracks or company dormitories, drug injectors may be living on the streets or in jail. None of these concentrations of people with risky behaviour will be picked up in a household survey, so the estimates based on the population prevalence may miss a significant number of people who are, in fact, part of the population of interest.

Thirdly, the more stigmatised a behaviour, the less likely people are to tell the truth about it to an interviewer, especially if they are approached in the context of their home and family. Household surveys therefore tend to give significant underestimates of the prevalence of very risky behaviours. The extent to which a behaviour is stigmatised clearly varies enormously by country.

In many Asian countries, male consumption of commercial sex is a cultural norm that carries little stigma, and household surveys have been used successfully to estimate the number of male clients of sex workers in several countries, including Thailand and Cambodia. On the other hand, it is unlikely in the Asian context that a household survey would yield good data about the much more marginalised practice of sex between men. In many Western countries, the reverse it true. Being gay is more socially acceptable than visiting sex workers. But even then, household surveys lead to underestimates.

In Canada, for example, the number of men who have sex with men was estimated from a general population survey reaching 2,500 people by telephone, as well as through three other indirect methods. In short, household surveys can serve to give a bare minimum estimate of stigmatised behaviours, but are unlikely to deliver the full picture in a cost-effective way. If a household survey is happening for another reason, however, it may be worth including questions about the behaviours of interest to get a minimum benchmark nationally, and then conduct special indepth validations in a smaller area to provide an estimate of the extent to which people are under-reporting the risky behaviour.

Multiplier methods generally rely on having information from two sources that overlap in a known way: the first is usually an institution or service with which the population to be estimated is in contact, and the second is the population at risk itself. Estimates are derived by multiplying the number of people who attend the institution or service over a certain period by the inverse of the proportion of the population who say they attended over the same period. Multiplier methods can also be used with information from two separate population-based survey samples that intersect in some way, as long as the size of one of the groups is relatively well known.

The most common example is sex workers and clients. In considering whether multiplier methods are appropriate, it is worth casting the net wide for potential sources of information. With a little planning even sources that are not immediately related to the behaviour in question can be used to arrive at estimates of sub-populations at risk for HIV. The good and the bad multiplier methods are relatively straightforward to use. They require good institutional record-keeping, and the right questions inserted into regular behavioural surveillance instruments. They are perhaps the most commonly used of all the population size estimation methods, and are very commonly found in economic and demographic literature.

However very few examples of the use of multiplier methods in estimating populations at risk for HIV have been recorded in the scientific "literature". This is probably precisely because they are simple and user-friendly. The greatest difficulty in using multiplier methods correctly is finding data for institutions and populations that correspond with one another. To use institutional and survey data together to estimate the size of a population, the members of the population all have to have a chance of being included in both the survey and in the institutional data.

One key issue in using multiplier methods successfully is the need to have clear, consistent definitions between different data sources. Firstly, the population definitions must be clear. In principle, it ought to be possible to use the proportion of drug users imprisoned together with the number of drug users in prison to arrive at an estimate of the number of drug users in a city or country.

Secondly, the time reference period must be clear, and must be the same in both data sources. Say you have a population based survey which asks men if they have visited sex workers in the last year: this would immediately give an estimate of the number of clients of sex workers.

Capture-recapture methods originated among naturalists trying to estimate the size of animal populations. A number of animals are captured, tagged and released. An independent recapture is conducted at a later time in the same area, and the proportion of the captured animals that have already been tagged is calculated. Information on the size of both captures and the proportion captured twice is entered into a mathematical formula to calculate the total size of the population, including the "unseen" portion.

Capture-recapture became fashionable in the early 1990s, and there was a rash of publications on its use in estimating the size of populations at risk for HIV around 1994. Since then, it has rather faded from view, for good reason. Capture-recapture techniques are useful in estimating the size of relatively hidden populations that are, none the less, in regular contact with two types of institutions or services.

One attempt at capture-recapture estimates compared individuals in treatment with individuals "captured" in police stations. However even here, the second "capture" was uncertain, since many drug users in detention are detained for offences not directly related to drug use. The principle of the independence of samples is frequently violated because institutions and services either cross-refer to one another or are mutually exclusive. Many possible entry points provide preferential access to one social class or another, and there may be important geographical variations.

A positive correlation will lead to an underestimate of the true population size, because it will increase the number of double-captures and therefore increase the size of the denominator for the population size calculation. A negative correlation, on the other hand, will lead to an overestimate of the entire population size, because the denominator (the number of dual-captures) will be smaller than would be expected if the samples were independent.

In some cases, a significant proportion of the overall population of interest has virtually no chance at all of ending up in either one of the "captures" and will therefore go unestimated. Sex workers who work by mobile phone and who serve the high end of the market will never be arrested, nor will they ever go to an STI screening and treatment centre in a red light district, even though their behaviour may still mean they are at high risk for HIV, for example.

As for the "integrity of the mark", that too is problematic. The most commonly used "mark" is the name, which appears on registers of those in treatment, in detention, etc. In some cultures, the pool of surnames is relatively small and it is difficult to distinguish between duplicates and separate individuals who have the same name. In some countries people regularly change names according to life events or because a new name may be associated with a change in fortune. Further, names may be spelt differently, and people may use different parts of their names in different situations.

On top of that, where illegal behaviours are concerned, people often give false names or aliases, which are not constant over time. Where the "mark" is a token given out during direct contact, different difficulties arise. If the token is of little value, people may forget having received it. If it is of significant value and more memorable, they may deny having received it in the hope of receiving another.

Capture-recapture techniques are only really reliable in "closed" populations, where there is no major inflow or outflow of people. Some of the sub-populations at high risk for HIV are peculiarly mobile. High migration rates undermine the ability to perform good capture-recapture. Equally, it is hard to use these methods when the population itself is changing rapidly, as is often the case in the early phases of an epidemic of drug injection, when large numbers of new injectors are constantly being recruited. Where data sources allow, these problems can be minimised by ensuring that two rounds of "capture" are as close together as possible in time.

REFERENCES

Auvert B, et al., "Ecological and individual level analysis of risk factors for HIV infection in four urban populations in sub-Saharan Africa with different levels of HIV infection". *AIDS*; 15: S15–30, 2001.

Dodds J., et al., "Increase in high-risk sexual behaviour among homosexual men", London 1996–8: crosssectional, questionnaire study, *British Medical Journal*; 320: 1510–1511, 2001.

Family Health International et al., "What drives HIV in Asia? A summary of trends in sexual and drug-taking behaviours", Arlington: *Family Health International*, 2001.

Monitoring the AIDS Pandemic (MAP), "The Status and Trends of HIV/AIDS/STI Epidemics in Asia and the Pacific". Provisional Report. Melbourne, 2001.

UNAIDS, *AIDS Epidemic Update 2001*, Geneva, 2001.

2

HIV: Challenges for Development

HIV/AIDS has become one of the most important challenges to the continued development of many countries in the world. The epidemic has wiped out four decades of development progress in the hardest hit countries. It is having a disproportionate effect on the poor and is, itself, massively exacerbated by poverty. Unless rapidly and effectively addressed, it will prevent the attainment of the health, education, and poverty reduction—the Millennium Development Goals target.

AIDS not only causes great human suffering but also, in the hardest hit countries, jeopardises economic growth and social and political stability. In sub Saharan Africa the epidemic is shattering families and placing extraordinary burdens on the extended family and village systems that have been the backbone of African child-rearing tradition. In countries where prevalence is lower, the impact on many highly vulnerable groups will be severe. The levels of infection are currently accelerating in India, South-East Asia, and the Newly Independent States. It is estimated that by 2005, more than 100 million people worldwide will be HIV-positive.

In the absence of an effective vaccine (a vaccine will not be available for some years), responding to HIV/AIDS will require a complex and long term commitment. Responses will vary from country to country, but the priority will be strategies to promote prevention, whilst reducing the impact of HIV/AIDS. Scaling up the response in the light of weak national capacity will require national, regional and sub-regional action. The solution to the epidemic lies in the development and implementation of comprehensive national responses, as described below, supported with adequate resources. Where formal systems are overwhelmed by the epidemic, greater importance will be placed on supporting communities to develop their own response, and finding ways to channel resources to them.

Table 1. Global estimates for the epidemic (end-2000)

Epidemiology		
	People living with HIV/AIDS	36.1m
	Deaths due to HIV/AIDS in 2000	3.0m
	Cumulative deaths due to HIV/AIDS	21.8m
Impact		
	Life expectancy reduced by up to 20–30 years	
	15.8 million AIDS orphans (30.2 million by 2010)	
	New HIV infections in 2000 5.3m	
	Negative population growth in 3 African countries	
	1–2 per cent loss in GDP per year in hardest hit countries since start of epidemic.	

Understanding HIV/AIDS: risk, vulnerability and impact.

Epidemiological Risk

HIV/AIDS has many interconnected causes and consequences. Any strategic response to the epidemic must be rooted in an understanding of why individuals are at risk of infection. The patterns of transmission and the relative importance of underlying factors will vary by country. Table 2 shows the principle means of transmission of the HIV virus.

The risk of sexual transmission of HIV is substantially increased by the presence of other sexually transmitted infections (STI), high rates of partner exchange, lack of health information, and the unavailability of condoms. The perception of risk in the future (as with smoking) is low in young people. It is closely related to self-esteem. Alcohol is associated with high risk behaviour in men.

Table 2: Proportion of HIV transmission globally

Per cent	*Means of transmission*
80	Sexual transmission (both heterosexual and homosexual)
5	Injecting drug use (sharing needles for injecting drug use)
5	Unsafe blood transfusions
10	Mother to child transmission (occurs *in utero*, during delivery and through breast-feeding).

Source: USAID

Women's frequent inability to negotiate sex and the use of condoms is a key factor. Moreover, biologically, women are five times more likely than men to be infected sexually. Women in particular, but also men, who only have one sexual partner are at risk should their partner have multiple other partners. Women with female genital mutilation may be at increased risk of HIV infection. Male circumcision is associated with a significant reduction in risk or transmission.

There are two main virus types, HIV-1 and HIV-2. HIV-1 is more easily transmissible than HIV-2 and contributes more heavily to the global pandemic. Ten different HIV-1 virus subtypes (or clades) have been identified as well as five HIV-2 clades. This poses substantial technical problems for vaccine development.

The time between infection with HIV and death varies: it can be more than 10 years, but in developing countries is frequently less. "AIDS" refers to a clinical definition of when an individual's immune systems have become progressively weak. In developing countries, technology and systems do not exist to monitor population's immune systems. Anti-retroviral (ARV) therapies can delay the onset of full blown AIDS, but there is not sufficient evidence to show that they can also reduce transmission of HIV.

There is currently no effective vaccine against HIV. The first candidate vaccines are being tested on humans. It is estimated that effective vaccines could become available in about 10 years, and even when available will not be 100 per cent effective, so wider prevention work will still be necessary. There is not yet an effective vaginal microbicide suitable to prevent HIV transmission.

VULNERABILITY TO HIV INFECTION

Vulnerability to HIV infection and its consequences is determined by a complex set of interactions between a number of key factors. Effective responses depend on these factors being understood and appropriately addressed. Individuals and communities are most at risk when capabilities to avoid infection and deal adequately with its consequences are compromised by inequalities, discrimination, and failures of public policy.

Many factors impact on vulnerability. These include the following:

— Gender inequalities make women and girls particularly vulnerable because they are often compromised in their ability to negotiate safe sex or to ward off unwanted sexual attention.

— The vulnerability of young people is increased significantly if they are deprived of information and reproductive health, education, and other services. The vulnerability of refugees and migrants can be increased by similar factors.

— Discrimination against people living with HIV and AIDS, and those who care for them, multiplies the burden of care on family and friends and excludes infected people from adequate support and treatment.

— Inadequate or inappropriate public information, and the absence of counselling and support services, reduce people's capacities to protect themselves from infection and behave responsibly towards others.

— Fear of stigma and discrimination discourages people from seeking counselling and support where this is available, and increases the likelihood that infection will be passed to others.

— Heavy-handed responses to commercial sex and drug use and to homosexuality can lead to exclusion from counselling and information and adequate health services, and initiatives such as condom supply and needle exchange programmes, and thus increase the risks of transmission.

— Poverty, insecure livelihoods, and lack of social protection can increase the likelihood of risky behaviour and undermine capacities to cope with the consequences of infection, creating downward spirals in both vulnerabilities to infection and its consequences.

Preventing the spread of HIV/AIDS, and coping with its impact is particularly difficult during emergencies and conflict situations. Prevention and care facilities and social networks break down along with social services and infrastructure. Increased population migration, the particular living conditions in refugee camps, and the breakdown of norms and values that govern sexual behaviour can all contribute to increased spread of the virus and the onset of AIDS. Armed forces can show particularly high HIV infection rates compared to civilians and their contact with local populations and the sex industries that tend to grow up around them can increase the spread of HIV.

IMPACT OF HIV/AIDS EPIDEMIC ON DEVELOPMENT

More than 95 per cent of HIV infected people live in the developing world. HIV/AIDS is reversing life expectancy gains made in the last 40 years. By 2000 life expectancy had declined by 20-30 years in the hardest hit countries. Population structures are also being radically altered. The economically active age group of 15-45 year olds are particularly severely hit.

In Botswana in 20 years time there will be more adults in their 60s and 70s than in their 40s and 50s.

The epidemic has increased mortality rates and now threatens the child and maternal international development targets; 55 per cent of HIV positive adults in sub-Saharan Africa are women and at the end of 2000 there were 1.4 million children living with HIV/AIDS. Women and children also bear a heavy burden of coping with the impact of HIV in families.

There is growing evidence that high HIV prevalence is linked with reduced gross domestic product (GDP). UNAIDS estimate that as HIV prevalence rises to 20 per cent or more, GDP growth may decline by up to 2 per cent per year. In South Africa HIV/AIDS is projected to reduce the economic growth rate by 0.3 – 0.4 per cent annually, resulting in the GDP in 2010 being 17 per cent lower than it would have been without AIDS.

The epidemic contributes to skills shortages in a shrinking labour force, weakens incentives for investment and strains government budgets. HIV/AIDS reduces the productivity and profitability of businesses and enterprises. Worker absenteeism due to illness and funeral attendance reduces productivity. Employer covered burial and health care costs, increasingly high labour turnover, and increased staff training costs, combine to reduce profitability.

In many countries, especially sub-Saharan Africa, HIV/AIDS is putting an enormous strain on health and education services by drastically reducing the number of staff, the number of new trainees, and the length of service of current staff with HIV/AIDS. The institutional capacity of services is being seriously affected. At the same time the health care sector is overwhelmed with a massive increase in patients (up to 80 per cent of hospital beds being occupied by HIV related illness). In addition there is evidence of declining school attendance rates, in particular of girls, as children assume caring or head of household roles, supporting or replacing parents with HIV/AIDS.

HIV/AIDS has a major impact on the households of people living with the disease. Households are driven to develop short-term coping strategies which tend to have negative long term consequences as, for example, young girls miss school to take on caring responsibilities. HIV/AIDS impacts on the food and livelihood security of households and communities.

Households' financial and non-financial assets are threatened by illness and death. Human capital diminishes as people and skills are lost and social networks break down. Physical capital is depleted as farmland becomes poorly managed. As livelihoods are threatened and productivity undermined, nutrition and health declines.

In rural settings, poor people's vulnerability will depend on their wider capacity to manage the impact of HIV/AIDS on the household. This will be dependent not only on labour, physical and non-physical assets and markets, but also on mitigating the stigma that HIV imposes in such communities.

In 2000, the UN Security Council acknowledged HIV/AIDS as a global security risk as well as a human security issue. The high attrition caused by AIDS deaths in the armed forces and police of many sub-Saharan African countries risks exacerbating instability. The spread of HIV can increase as armies with high HIV prevalence are involved in peacekeeping activities in other countries. And, high HIV prevalence and the subsequent socioeconomic impact on societies can be politically destabilising.

Failure to control AIDS is an index of inequitable development and poor governance. Income inequality, gender inequality, labour migration, conflict and refugee movement all promote the spread of HIV. Despite the widely recognised benefits of globalisation, more than a billion of the world's 6 billion people still cannot fulfil their basic needs for food, water, sanitation, health care, housing and education. Worldwide, an estimated 1.1 billion people are malnourished. An estimated 1.2 billion people live on less than US$1 a day. In more than 30 of the poorest national economies (most of them in sub-

Saharan Africa), real per capita incomes have been declining since the early 1980s. At the same time, pressures on States to provide basic services and infrastructure have not eased. The HIV/AIDS epidemic, along with other diseases, conflicts and droughts, is worsening matters further.

But the global response to AIDS shows that the negative effects of globalisation need not be 'facts of life'. Greater access to high income countries' markets, debt relief and more development aid will go a long way towards enabling countries to reduce poverty. High-income countries spent more than US$300 billion in 2001 on agricultural subsidies—roughly equivalent to the combined gross domestic product of all of sub-Saharan Africa. It is clear that AIDS represents a long and devastating tale of exclusion for millions of people, with or without HIV infection.

The expanding AIDS epidemic provides a compelling case for accelerating much-needed global reform in an effort to better support local responses. This can be done by: creating stronger international cooperation, guided by the principles of human rights; generating more accountability and transparency of international institutions; replenishing national capabilities to safeguard the right to health (including the provision of HIV prevention, access to HIV care or the development of a HIV vaccine), and enlisting the help of the business sector in such efforts; redressing global poverty (a driving force of the AIDS epidemic) by, among other things, increasing Official Development Assistance to at least 0.7 per cent of gross national product (a level first agreed to by the international community in 1969 and since endorsed repeatedly, including at the 2002 Monterrey International Conference on Financing for Development); and above all, setting new rules of the game to ensure a more equitable distribution of the fruits of globalisation.

The world cannot afford to wait until the perfect conditions exist before acting against AIDS. The fight against AIDS cannot go on hold until human security is achieved and poverty is eliminated. The growing global response to AIDS needs to be bolstered by stronger human security, equality and justice. In the long run, success in the struggle against the epidemic requires a global community that acts on the basis of human concern and humane values.

TACKLING HIV/AIDS

HIV/AIDS is a communicable disease driven by the behaviour of individuals. As a result, no one intervention is the key to success. We have learnt much about what needs to be done to tackle the epidemic.

The important elements in tackling HIV/AIDS are:

- Political commitment and leadership at all levels;
- Sustained effort over a long period of time;
- Effective global and national surveillance;
- National resource mobilisation – Uganda:
- $2 per capita/year from the national budget;
- National capacity building across all sectors for a broad based response;
- Policies and programmes which tackle the locally specific epidemic;
- Early action in low prevalence countries;
- Mobilisation of civil society, private sector and faith based organisations;
- Willingness to deal with stigma and discrimination.

Not all of these elements have always been in place, but the key message is clear: with a combination of these it is possible to tackle HIV/AIDS. Thailand has done just that with strong government support, resources and focused interventions. Some countries have successfully reduced the rate of new HIV cases or maintained low levels of prevalence over time either by preventing a major epidemic (Senegal with STI control, Thailand with condoms) or by reducing an existing severe epidemic (Uganda, Thailand, Zambia, Dominican Republic). Prevention alone cannot succeed. Incorporation of a prevention to care continuum is required to ensure that persons living with HIV/AIDS receive appropriate care. These individuals, in turn, often become the best change agents for prevention.

Reducing the Risk of Infection

There are a limited number of interventions that can reduce sexual transmission of HIV. STD treatment, condoms, and voluntary counselling and testing (VCT) are effective, particularly when targeted to high HIV prevalent populations and to couples. VCT is even more effective when linked to care and support services.

Interventions that work to prevent sexual transmission include:

— Male and female condoms are the only reliable barrier method.

— Combinations of strategies to deliver condoms are necessary to cover areas of wide geographical and socio-economic diversity, including free and subsidised provision through health services and social marketing.

— Behaviour change programmes are an essential and effective part of strategies to reduce high risk behaviour.

— Voluntary Counselling and Testing (VCT) for HIV is vital to enable people to make decisions about their behaviour based upon accurate knowledge of their, or their sexual partners, HIV status.

— Improved diagnosis and management of other STIs reduces the risk of HIV transmission.

Injecting drug use. An open and tolerant legislative regime that works with drug users helps reduce HIV transmission through injecting drug use. Programmes can include needle exchange provision, methadone treatment facilities, information and education campaigns that promote needle and syringe disinfecting techniques and reduce sharing of needles. Attempts to change sexual risk behaviour of injecting drug users have been less successful.

Blood safety. Ensuring the safety of blood transfusions and blood products in developing countries reduces HIV and other blood born infections (hepatitis, malaria) and increases confidence in health services. Interventions that can improve the safety of blood include selective recruitment of voluntary blood donors (such as focusing on youth), screening of blood donations and substituting the use of blood with alternative methods.

Mother to child transmission (MTCT). Approximately a third of infants born to mothers with HIV are HIV positive. ARV reduces the risk of mother to child transmission by up to 50 per cent. WHO recommends the provision of nevirapine, a low cost ARV, to reduce MTCT. There are complex issues surrounding MTCT involving infant feeding, treatment for the mother, and health system support needs.

Reducing Vulnerability

The key to reducing vulnerability is to create an environment that enables people, both women and men, to access and use the interventions outlined above. To achieve this requires strong and sustained political commitment. Government and civil society need to open out the public discussion about HIV/AIDS, sex, and gender relations and promote openness and respect for the human rights of all people. Explicit commitment to tackling stigma and discrimination is essential. Participatory models can help identify how best to support the most vulnerable, and develop strategies to provide them with the information they need.

The societies which have been most successful in facing the challenge of HIV/AIDS have been those in which it has been faced openly, and where communities of support have been built for, and by, those at risk and those affected. Strong leadership is required to bring the debate about HIV/AIDS out into the open, and to create a supportive policy and legal framework and to challenge social norms which increase vulnerability. Civil society must embrace people living with HIV and AIDS and create an atmosphere of active support and social inclusion. The rights of all people to control their own sex lives and demand safe sex must be actively upheld.

Information about all aspects of HIV/AIDS must be freely and widely available, and public debate stimulated and encouraged and led from the highest levels.

Mass media campaigns, using appropriate communication strategies and locally appropriate idioms, are an essential element. Top-down information campaigns are rarely as effective as more interactive media such as soap opera and theatre, where complex issues and differing views and perspectives can be fully explored and public debate encouraged. Peer-based support and dialogue, among youth and other at-risk groups including long distance transport workers, is also important.

Effective education programmes raise awareness of actual risk of infection. Ensuring people's rights to information and training programmes helps women and girls negotiate condom use with sexual partners and to delay their first sexual contact. Behaviour change, and other communication programmes, supported by a positive policy environment, can be an effective part of HIV control strategies and should be properly integrated into national HIV/AIDS control programmes. They need a coordinated approach to communications involving government, local and national media and civil society.

HIV/AIDS is causing unprecedented human resource loss in education systems. Ministries of Education and Labour need to develop and implement strategies to prevent severe skill shortages in both the public and private sector. This can include investigating new pathways into education, distance learning methodologies, access to training and education and in the longer term the expansion of training facilities and their throughput.

Education helps prevent the spread of HIV and build a society which reduces stigma and accepts persons living with HIV/AIDS (PLWHA). Education plays an important role in achieving difficult changes in societal norms. Focusing on children and youth is an effective part of this. The young, especially pre-sexually active youth and children, are more open to behavioural change initiatives. Young people, females in particular, are particularly vulnerable.

Social protection of the most vulnerable, especially women and children, helps give them more control over their lives, and reduces their vulnerability, for example, by ensuring that children are not forced into unequal sexual relations with adults. Access to wider economic opportunities can reduce the vulnerability of poor people to exploitation, and reduce vulnerability to risky behaviour. In some cases, income generating schemes and wider livelihood opportunities can provide alternatives to commercial sex work.

We have a lot to learn from existing reproductive health programmes. Long-term commitment from government and the international community is essential. In Bangladesh, a remarkable success story, it took 15 years of sustained political and donor commitment to develop an open family planning programme leading to more than 50 per cent of couples currently using effective family planning methods.

Treatment and Care

The long term development of stronger, pro-poor, sustainable health systems is essential to ensuring the safe delivery of treatment and care for HIV/AIDS. Services for addressing HIV/AIDS need to be fully integrated into health services as they strengthen and extend their coverage. Treatment involves clinical interventions ranging from addressing opportunistic infections such as TB to provision of ARV therapy. With 40 per cent of AIDS deaths due to TB, treatment can have significant effects on length and quality of life.

The ultimate aim is to maintain the best possible quality of life for as long as possible for persons living with HIV/AIDS without bankrupting the family. Developing a prevention-care continuum, which maximises community and home-based care and treatment, improves the quality of life of PLWHA and reduces the burden on their families.

Counselling for individuals and families is an essential part of any minimum package of care. Many families of PLWHA, as with all marginal and vulnerable groups, need support to ensure food security and good shelter while coping as part of broader strategies to ensure their livelihoods.

Anti-retrovirals (ARV)

Anti-retrovirals are becoming less expensive, offering hope to many people, but they are still unaffordable to most poor people. There are significant equity, cost and sustainability issues. ARVs must be taken for life and are highly toxic drugs. Even if they were free, it is not feasible for health systems in many poor countries to deliver these drugs safely and equitably. Until safe and equitable systems can be put in place it would be inappropriate to use scarce resources to support widescale provision of ARVs for treatment.

Monitoring and Evaluation

Trends in the epidemic vary between countries as does the profile of those infected. In Russia HIV transmission is mostly due to injecting drug use and is high amongst commercial sex workers. In Africa heterosexual transmission is the predominant mode. Epidemiological data on key modes of transmission is necessary to guide the response to the epidemic and evaluate effectiveness of interventions. In particular the possible spread of transmission from high risk behaviour to the general population needs monitoring.

High quality epidemiological data is required to effectively guide policy to address the predominant mode of transmission. Worldwide, better data is required to measure the effectiveness of HIV/AIDS control programmes and their contribution towards the decline in new infection. It is important to distinguish whether plateaus in new cases are a result of successful control campaigns or because of natural containment of the epidemic among high-risk behaviour groups only.

Strategies to Protect the Next Generation

Strategies to reduce the impact of the epidemic can be targeted at individuals or across society. In many countries, the large number of orphans surviving the epidemic requires a concerted response, which aims to give them the best possible livelihood opportunities. Fostering is important but care is needed to ensure so far as possible that the children receive the same education, nutrition, and opportunities as children not orphaned by AIDS.

Community-based care is the only affordable care in most settings. Strategies to reduce impact should also address livelihood protection for households affected by AIDS related illness and death. These interventions may include micro-credits for people living with HIV/AIDS to help them sustain a livelihood.

The importance of education for development and health, in particular of female education is so great that the current threat to the education of children resulting from HIV/AIDS in many countries needs to be urgently addressed. Education is key to reducing impact, reducing future vulnerability, and ensuring that future renewal of skilled labour force occurs.

It is essential for all sectors of society and the economy to plan for a future with a drastically reduced skilled and unskilled labour force. Education, health, police, military, law enforcement, business and industry are already suffering from loss of skilled labour, the costs of recruiting and training new staff, and the cost of caring for current staff with HIV/AIDS.

Some companies have introduced employment-based health insurance to protect against the risk of infection, sexual health services (including for sex workers near major enterprises with residential workforces), and provision of care and counselling. Some large companies in West Africa even provide ARVs, judging that their provision outweighs the costs of loss of skilled staff.

There is considerable ongoing research into the impact of HIV/AIDS, the effects of policy responses, effective approaches to HIV/AIDS prevention and on new technologies to prevent HIV transmission and treat HIV/AIDS. Vaccine research needs to focus on the clades that are most prevalent in developing countries, as immune response may be clade specific. The potential of vaginal microbicides as a female controlled means to prevention requires considerable attention.

Role of Governments and Civil Society

The fight against HIV/AIDS can only be won at the country level and with national leadership. Civil society also provides valuable leadership, both with government and in many countries where government has not yet responded to the epidemic. The variability in prevalence of the epidemic requires governments to develop different strategies, even within the same country. A range of activities can be recommended for the different stages of the epidemic which countries or provinces can undertake.

Key elements of successful national response are:

- — HIV/AIDS fully recognised and addressed within HIPC, PRSP, UNDAF and SWAP processes, and national responses are multisectoral and are sustainably embedded with the national budget.
- — All sectors plan to reduce the impact of the epidemic.
- — Addressing the underlying causes of vulnerability, in particular human rights, stigma, discrimination and gender inequalities.
- — Support is provided to ensure that the education system is suitably harnessed to address HIV/AIDS prevention and

manage the impact of AIDS on schools and educational institutions.

— Support, including resources, through the public and private sector is provided to ensure that condoms are fully accessible.

— Working with civil society and NGOs to maximise their contribution.

— Capacity is built to enable countries to deliver high quality prevention, treatment and care for PLWHA. This will require substantially strengthened health systems.

— Monitoring and surveillance systems are developed to measure effectiveness and guide priority setting.

International agencies have important roles to play in generating global political commitment and supporting effective, coordinated action at country level. UNAIDS has an important role in advocacy, resource mobilisation and providing global leadership. The United Nations General Assembly Special Session on HIV/AIDS in June 2001 should catalyse an intensified international effort to provide better support for countries to effectively fight HIV/AIDS.

WHO has a key role as the global normative technical agency. It needs to improve its own support to countries and increase its capacity to address HIV/AIDS. Other UNAIDS cosponsors also have important global responsibilities: UNICEF on MTCT and education issues, UNFPA on ensuring long-term global contraceptive security, and the World Bank on resource mobilisation, policy dialogue and programme implementation with countries.

Civil society and in particular non-governmental organisations (NGOs) play a vital role in combating HIV/AIDS. Their strengths include advocating on behalf of PLWHA, addressing stigma, creating an environment of openness, advocating human rights, and in particular tackling gender inequalities. Civil society organisations are most able to work with vulnerable groups, with NGOs providing prevention and care for high-risk groups including men who have sex with men and sex workers. NGOs have a role in care and treatment for PLWHA and in voluntary counselling and testing.

REFERENCES

Bloom D. et al., *Health, wealth, AIDS and Poverty*, Cambridge: Harvard School of Public Health, 2002.

Bollinger L., Stover J., *The Economic Impact of AIDS*, Washington: The Futures Group International, 1999.

Hecht R., *Poverty, debt and AIDS—mainstreaming the epidemic and mobilising additional resources for the response*, Geneva, UNAIDS, Inter-Country Team for West and Central Africa, 2000.

Hecht R, Adeyi O., Semini I., "Making AIDS Part of the Global Development Agenda", *Finance & Development*: 39(1). Washington: IMF, 2002.

Loewenson R., Whiteside A. *HIV/AIDS. Implications for poverty reduction*, New York, UNDP, 2001.

UNAIDS, *A Multi-Ministerial Strategy to the Expanded Response to HIV/AIDS. HIV/AIDS Development in Asia and the Pacific: A lengthening shadow*, Geneva. 2001.

_______________ , *A strategic approach towards an AIDS-competent society. Local responses to HIV/AIDS*, Geneva, 2001.

UNDP, Human Development Report, 2001. New York, 2001.

UNICEF, *The epidemiology of HIV at the start of the 21st century*, New York, 2002.

United Nations General Assembly, *Declaration of Commitment on HIV/AIDS: 'Global Crisis—Global Action*. 2001.

Webb D., Elliott L., *Learning to Live: Monitoring and evaluating HIV/AIDS programmes for young people*, London: Save the Children/Department for International Development/UNAIDS. 2000.

World Bank, *World Development Report 2000/2001: Attacking poverty*, Washington, 2001.

3

HIV/AIDS and Human Rights

HIV/AIDS is a human rights catastrophe. The epidemic has emerged as the single greatest threat to the fulfilment of the rights of children and women in all over the world. Those affected are routinely denied their rights to education, economic opportunity and health care and to protection from exploitation and harm. They are discriminated against and left powerless to resist the dangers they face. Yet every government has a responsibility to create an environment where children's rights are protected and defended.

Almost every country in the world has ratified the Convention on the Rights of the Child (CRC), which recognises that children have the right to develop to their fullest potential physically, mentally and socially, and to express their opinions freely. The cost of HIV/AIDS rises with each minute the epidemic grows. As HIV/AIDS spreads, the cost of tackling the epidemic increases. In affected countries, trends in reducing child mortality and malnutrition and in expanding access to education are being reversed; and the population of orphans and other vulnerable children is exploding.

The potential of young people to develop, and to participate in and contribute to society is being threatened as HIV/AIDS kills their mothers and fathers, brothers and sisters, schoolteachers, friends and young people themselves. Guided by the principles of the CRC and the Convention on the Elimination of All Forms of Discrimination against Women (CEDAW), UNICEF will over the next several years focus its efforts on HIV/AIDS as one of five priority areas of action where the potential for change and impact on children's lives is considered to be the greatest. The other four priorities are girls' education; early childhood; immunisation 'plus' strengthening health systems; and protecting children from violence, abuse, exploitation and discrimination.

Around the world, the risk for girls and women of contracting HIV is compounded by their generally low economic and social status and by pervasive gender discrimination. Girls and women are often denied access to critical information, education and knowledge about sexuality and how to protect themselves from HIV/AIDS. They often lack the power to say no to sex both within and outside of marriage, to choose their own partners and to influence sexual behaviour.

Widows are often denied their rights and property, an injustice that can force them and their children into exploitative situations, dramatically increasing their risk for contracting HIV. And during civil unrest and armed conflict, young women and girls are even more likely to become victims of sexual violence and coercion. This pervasive denial of basic human rights is deadly.

In some countries, HIV prevalence among teenage girls is five times higher than among teenage boys. Most of these infections occur as a result of unprotected heterosexual sex, often with older men. The danger of infection is highest among the poorest and least powerful. Young people who inject drugs, are affected by armed conflict, suffer sexual exploitation, or live on the streets or in institutions have even less access to information, skills, services and support than young people normally do.

HIV/AIDS arises from and exacerbates many of the interlocking problems that affect children, including poverty, malnutrition, discrimination, inadequate access to basic services, armed conflict, gender inequities and the sexual exploitation of girls and women. At the same time, the pandemic overstretches and depletes the capacities of government services, communities and families to ensure the protection and fulfilment of children's rights in the face of these challenges.

UNICEF has expanded its support to programmes working with young people to inform them about HIV/AIDS, develop their life skills, encourage them to adopt healthy and safer behaviours, and increase their access to youth-friendly health services. Prevention of mother-to-child transmission of HIV has also been expanded. UNICEF has also collaborated closely with fellow UNAIDS co-sponsors and with bilateral and multilateral organisations.

UNICEF is committed to an aggressive response to HIV/AIDS not only because of the extraordinary threat posed by AIDS to children, but also because HIV infection is preventable. Throughout the world, families and communities are successfully confronting the epidemic. These successes, however, have remained limited and small in scale. Therefore, the principal challenge in the medium term is to mobilise the leadership, partnerships, participation and resources to ensure the intensity and coverage of efforts needed to halt new infections and to provide care and support for those struggling with HIV and AIDS.

More specifically, UNICEF will support actions to:

i) prevent new infections among young people;
ii) prevent parent-to-child transmission of HIV;
iii) expand access to care and support for children and their families living with HIV and AIDS; and
iv) ensure care, protection and support for children orphaned or otherwise made vulnerable by AIDS.

In the midst of conflict, UNICEF must ensure that the humanitarian response addresses HIV/AIDS. Conflict creates and exacerbates the conditions—and human rights abuses—in which HIV/AIDS flourishes. These conditions include the disintegration of communities, displacement, the separation of children from their families, rape and other sexual violence, and the destruction of schools and health services.

At the same time, women and girls are often left so destitute that, for many, trading sex for money becomes their only survival option. Without addressing these conditions, HIV/AIDS-prevention activities in emergency situations cannot be effective. Due to these factors, UNICEF's priorities in fighting HIV/AIDS in conflict areas differ from those in stable settings. These priorities are to:

i) assess and analyse the extent and causes of children's and young people's vulnerability to HIV/AIDS, particularly that caused by displacement, sexual violence, lack of protection, and economic desperation;
ii) advocate for the protection of children and young people from sexual violence and exploitation and for the provision of information, education and services to prevent HIV infection;
iii) support the actions of governments, non-state entities, NGOs, civil society and community organisations to prevent and respond to sexual violence and exploitation; inform young people about HIV and how to prevent it and ensure their access to essential health services, including provision of condoms and treatment for sexually transmitted infections (STIs); and ensure protection and care for orphans and children separated from their families; and
iv) monitor the effectiveness of actions.

Human rights guide all programme processes at UNICEF, including how the organisation assesses and analyses the situation of children and women; how it designs and supports programmes; how it builds partnerships and alliances with and for children and young people; and how it develops strategies to influence public policy and resource allocation. A human rights approach recognises that children and young people are 'rights holders' and that States, governments, parents and other adults are obliged, in various ways, to ensure the fulfilment of children's human rights, working with children in the process.

Building upon this relationship between 'rights holders' and those who are obliged to fulfil those rights, a human rights programming approach strengthens everyone's abilities to recognise rights violations and threats, and to understand their underlying causes. Through this approach UNICEF can better understand the extent to which families, communities, local governments and States have responded to these threats and violations as well as the factors preventing such action. On the basis of this analysis, a human rights programming approach is used to identify actions that will strengthen the capacities of individuals and groups to protect children's rights.

The importance of preventing HIV/AIDS cannot be overestimated, both in countries where HIV/AIDS is already established and in those where its threat is not yet widely felt. Typically, this programming process is undertaken by teams involving children, family and community members, and key government, NGO and civil society partners. It results in action plans that involve and are supported by a broad range of development partners. Implementation of these action plans is monitored, and adjustments are made based on the progress achieved and lessons learned.

At the country level the organisation will work towards achieving several goals: to strengthen the capacities of governments and their partners to assess and understand the HIV/AIDS epidemic in each situation and its impact on children; to assess the adequacy of current responses; and to design and implement programmes that expand the coverage and impact of actions to prevent HIV/AIDS and provide care for affected children, young people, and families.

Every country and region will have to refine and balance the corporate strategies outlined above in order to respond to its particular local situation. The first priority, for all countries, is to halt the epidemic or epidemics in their countries and reverse rising HIV incidence rates. This will require large-scale actions for preventing new infections—particularly among children and young people—in Eastern and Southern Africa, West and Central Africa, South and South-East Asia, the Caribbeans, Latin America, and Central and Eastern Europe.

The importance of preventing HIV/AIDS cannot be overestimated, both in countries where HIV/AIDS is already established and in those where its threat is not yet widely felt. In areas where HIV prevalence is relatively low or concentrated among particularly vulnerable groups, programmes are likely to have a dual focus: first, to promote the general healthy development of young people and thus prevent HIV infection; and second, to immediately address the needs of people most at risk of contracting the disease.

This is particularly important in countries with large populations vulnerable to HIV/AIDS. In all affected countries, the capacities of groups and individuals at all levels of government and civil society must be strengthened to care for people living with HIV/AIDS, orphans and other groups made vulnerable by the disease, and to address the medium- and longer-term development consequences. UNICEF will make HIV/AIDS a priority in all countries affected by HIV/AIDS.

HIV/AIDS AND INTERNATIONAL HUMAN RIGHTS LAW

The Joint United Nations Programme on HIV/AIDS (UNAIDS) estimated that AIDS had killed almost 25 million people between the beginning of the epidemic and the end of 2001, that another 40 million people were living with HIV/ AIDS by the end of 2001, and that five million new cases were diagnosed in 2001 alone. Young women, men who have sex with men, and injecting drug users are particularly vulnerable to infection with HIV. These groups are often characterised by social and economic disadvantage and discrimination; this leads to the observation that in each society, those people who before the arrival of HIV/AIDS were marginalised, stigmatised and discriminated against become over time those at highest risk of HIV infection.

The determinants, scope and impact of the global epidemic of HIV/AIDS in epidemiological, social and human terms have been substantially documented. We know how the virus is transmitted, the effectiveness of prevention strategies in individuals and populations and how to slow disease progression in those infected with the virus. Yet in almost all of the developing and transitional countries, where the majority of new cases are occurring, the response has been unable to stop and reverse the tide of infection. HIV/AIDS are now recognised as an immense challenge to international security, peace and development. The continued escalation of infection, particularly in Africa, needs a coherent social epidemiology that understands the epidemic in its historical, political and international legal context.

Human rights are a set of universal entitlements that individuals enjoy irrespective of their sex, nationality, religion, culture or other status, that are inherent to human beings and that are proclaimed and protected by international law. Human rights have major relevance for shaping appropriate responses to the HIV epidemic and other global health challenges, including offering system-wide public health responses and identifying deficiencies in public health research agendas.

International human rights law developed in the context of global revulsion at the horrors of the Second World War and the establishment of the United Nations (UN) in 1945. In accepting the Charter of the United Nations, its member states recognise that non-interference in their internal affairs is a principle that can be overriden where international peace and security are threatened. No doubt referring to the genocide and other war crimes of Nazi Germany, the drafters of the 1948 Universal Declaration of Human Rights were moved to refer to "disregard and contempt for human rights [which] have resulted in barbarous acts [that] have outraged the conscience of mankind ... ". Although the declaration is not in itself a legally binding document, it reiterates that "human rights should be protected by the rule of law".

Today, a growing body of international treaties and customary international law details the obligation of states to respect, protect and fulfil human rights. States party to the two major covenants, for example, must not only avoid abuses of civil and political rights by their own agents, they must also prevent private sector discrimination and other abuses, while also "taking steps, individually and through international assistance and co-operation, especially economic and technical, to the maximum of ... available resources, with a view to achieving progressively the full realisation" of economic, social and cultural rights, including the right to health. These obligations are as binding as any other international legal agreements on, for example, maritime law or the protection of intellectual property.

International human rights law and HIV/AIDS Jonathan Mann, the first Director of the World Health Organisation (WHO)'s Global Programme on AIDS, identified the international law of human rights as a comprehensive framework to which public health practitioners could anchor responsibility for addressing the underlying causes of HIV/AIDS, trauma and other threats to health. Such a 'rights-based approach' to public health in general, and HIV/AIDS in particular, supports sound public health practice by providing additional tools to motivate governments to act to achieve public health goals. Rights considerations can help facilitate the setting and monitoring of public health targets and provide a complementary language to identify failures, or incipient failures, of public health programmes.

The rights-based approach also provides links with other social movements that use the same language—for example, the women's movement, the struggles of indigenous peoples and the movement of people working to protect the environment. In 1996, an international expert consultation group convened by UNAIDS and the Office of the High Commissioner for

Human Rights, which included human rights experts, representatives of national AIDS programmes, people living with HIV/AIDS, and non-governmental organisations, prepared guidelines for states on the application of international human rights law in the context of HIV/AIDS.

The guidelines were included in the report of the consultation tabled at the 53rd session of the Commission on Human Rights in 1997. The Commission welcomed the report and invited states to consider the guidelines (now known as the International Guidelines on HIV/AIDS and Human Rights). Subsequent resolutions in 1999 and 2001 asked states to report on measures taken, where appropriate, to promote and implement these guidelines, and tools have been prepared to help specific groups implement the guidelines in their areas of responsibility.

The commentary that accompanies the guidelines addresses complex issues in areas such as confidentiality and disclosure of HIV status by applying international legal principles to these dilemmas. The guidelines note that the international law of human rights allows states to impose limitations on certain personal freedoms, such as the right to liberty of movement, but only where the state can establish that the restriction is:

- provided for and carried out in accordance with the law, i.e. according to specific legislation that is accessible, clear and precise, so that it is reasonably foreseeable that individuals will regulate their conduct accordingly;
- based on a legitimate interest, as defined in the provisions guaranteeing the rights;
- proportional to that interest and constituting the least intrusive and least restrictive measure available and actually achieving that interest in a democratic society, i.e., established in a decision-making process consistent with the rule of law.

For example, the guidelines envisage circumstances in which public health legislation might legitimately authorise health care professionals to inform their patients' sexual partners of the HIV status of the patients. By requiring strict legal processes for any limitations on the rights of people infected, however, the guidelines reflect the "public health rationale" for preventing discrimination against people living with HIV/AIDS. In 2002, the High Commission for Human Rights and UNAIDS held another international consultation to revise the sixth guideline, which addresses access to prevention, treatment, care and support.

The revised guidelines recommend that domestic legislation incorporates safeguards and flexibilities in international agreements, such as intellectual property agreements, to promote and ensure access to HIV/AIDS prevention, treatment, care and support for all. In addition to international human rights law, other international legal agreements also influence the spread and impact of HIV/AIDS. For example, the agreements of the World Trade Organisation (WTO)—such as those that regulate the terms of trade and other matters between its members— greatly influence national income and the distribution of income within and between countries, and hence influence the resources available to governments for effective prevention, treatment and care.

What makes public health sense does not automatically become a human rights obligation in international law. Thus international human rights law does not provide particular guidance on injecting drug use, other than the general principles of non-discrimination and the obligations to control diseases, which can arguably be used to require the introduction of proven public health measures such as needle and syringe programmes.

Although international human rights treaties include monitoring mechanisms, and some provide for individual complaints about states' behaviour, the provisions for enforcement are generally weak, unlike, for example, trade agreements. In contrast with WTO infringements, no mechanism exists to impose monetary fines on violators of human rights.

International human rights law, as reflected in the International Guidelines on HIV/AIDS and Human Rights, does not provide, or claim to provide, a moral code for living with HIV/AIDS. It says nothing, for example, about our personal moral responsibility to care for affected people, although it addresses states' obligations in these areas.

Historically, human rights approaches in Western countries have tended to privilege civil and political rights over socio-economic and developmental rights. In the early years of the epidemic, this prompted a focus on discrimination against people living with HIV/AIDS and on vulnerable groups, such as men who have sex with men, which reflected the preoccupations with individual rights and protection of citizens from state interference typical of American civil libertarianism.

For many developing countries, however, such a narrow concept of rights fails to engage with the full range of social, political and cultural factors that underlie vulnerability to HIV and responses to AIDS. It is not surprising, therefore, that practitioners in developing countries may be sceptical of approaches that focus solely on libertarian notions of rights. This reinforces the need for human rights approaches to policy development which are able to integrate attention to socio-economic rights in response to HIV. For public health practitioners, developing, using, evaluating and adapting planning tools that bring the full spectrum of human rights into mainstream public health policy are the ways to integrate these rights in day-to-day practice.

Human Rights Law in Mitigation of HIV/AIDS

United Nations General Assembly Declaration of Commitment on HIV/AIDS The United Nations General Assembly's Declaration of Commitment on HIV/AIDS notes that "the full realisation of human rights and fundamental freedoms for all is an essential element in a global response to the HIV/AIDS pandemic". It also sets concrete, timebound targets for the introduction of national legislation and other measures to ensure the respect of rights in regard to education, inheritance, employment, health care, social and health services, prevention, support, treatment, information and legal protection.

Although states are not legally bound to implement the promises made in the declaration, the General Assembly's annual review of states' progress in meeting these commitments and the monitoring instruments being developed to measure compliance provide powerful tools to encourage government action.

Global Fund for AIDS, Tuberculosis and Malaria, The Board of the Global Fund for AIDS, Tuberculosis and Malaria sought to promote dialogue and collaboration between government and civil society during the preparation of funding proposals by requiring demonstrated consultation with and participation of affected communities. Participation is key to the rights-based approach to development, although the Board may be more influenced by practical considerations than by legal considerations in this respect. Non-governmental representatives who sit on the Board and technical advisory committee can monitor governments that try to falsify their applications.

Following the global outcry about the high cost of drugs for the treatment of HIV/AIDS, including anti-retroviral drugs, the WTO's Ministerial Council declared in November 2001 that the agreement on Trade-Related Aspects of Intellectual Property Rights (the TRIPS agreement) "does not and should not prevent members from taking measures to protect public health". The WTO statement followed the decision by Brazil to allow the local generic manufacture of patented medications unless the manufacturers drastically reduced the cost of the drugs or started making them in Brazil. In June 2002, the TRIPS Council (the body responsible for administering the TRIPS agreement) postponed until 2006 the end of the transition period during which least-developed countries do not have to provide patent protection for pharmaceuticals.

In 1999, UNAIDS and the Inter-Parliamentary Union jointly published the Handbook for Legislators on HIV/AIDS, Law and Human Rights. In September 2001, the 106th Inter-Parliamentary Conference in Ouagadougou, Burkina Faso, called on all parliamentarians "to step up their national efforts to establish effective national and international AIDS policies and programmes ... including the use of condoms, measures to counter discrimination and the provision of care to affected persons, including orphans." The resolution urged governments to give human rights precedence over trade rights, and it urged pharmaceutical companies to reduce the prices of medicines "above all in developing countries".

In November 2001, UNAIDS convened an Expert Panel on HIV Testing in UN Peacekeeping Operations to discuss whether the UN should introduce mandatory HIV testing for peacekeeping forces. Amongst other documentation, the panel considered a detailed submission based on international human rights law and national precedent. The panel unanimously rejected mandatory testing; instead it endorsed voluntary HIV counselling and testing for UN peacekeeping operations.

The International Guidelines on HIV/AIDS and Human Rights propose that states, through political and financial support, ensure community consultation in all phases of HIV/AIDS policy design, programme implementation and evaluation. Again, participation is key, because without this "reality check", governments risk introducing laws and policies that increase rather than diminish inequity and discrimination, and hence increase HIV infection and associated harms. For example, some governments have proposed amending the criminal law without fully considering the potential costs and benefits in public health terms, particularly from a gender perspective.

The Kenyan Legal Task Force on Issues Relating to HIV/AIDS provides an example of a participatory process. In June 2001, the Honourable Amos Wako, Attorney-General of Kenya (and former member of the UN Human Rights Committee), convened the Legal Task Force on Issues Relating to HIV/AIDS to make recommendations to the government on a possible legal framework for responding to the HIV/AIDS epidemic in Kenya. The task force undertook public consultations around the country and, in July 2002, it launched its report and recommendations. The Attorney-General promised that new legislation would be in place before the end of 2002.

In April 2001, 39 pharmaceutical companies bowed to worldwide condemnation by abandoning court action against the South African Government over legislation that could be used to make essential drugs affordable for millions of South Africans. In this case, the Treatment Action Campaign supported the government with arguments based, in part, on international human rights law and obligations.

In July 2002, the Constitutional Court of South Africa held that the constitution required the government "to devise and implement within its available resources a comprehensive and coordinated programme to realise progressively the rights of pregnant women and their newborn children to have access to health services to combat mother-to-child transmission of HIV".

The human rights protections in the Constitution of South Africa were constructed to reflect international human rights laws that bound South Africa, and the Treatment Action Campaign argued, with evident success, that government policy was in breach of South Africa's international legal obligations. By introducing international human rights law into a popular and militant public health campaign, a growing social movement successfully achieved a major shift in a national policy on HIV.

Although less organised and less visible in popular mobilisation than Treatment Action Campaign, women's rights activists in South Africa effectively used human rights arguments drawn from international law to influence the formulation of national policies relating to key areas of women's vulnerability to HIV, including domestic violence, sex discrimination and reproductive health rights. Such strategies are beginning to permeate the Southern African region.

In 1999, the Australian National Council on AIDS and Related Diseases published an instrument to measure states' compliance with the International Guidelines on HIV/AIDS and Human Rights. In July 2001, the UK All-Party Parliamentary Group on AIDS published a report of the inquiry into the UK's respect for and promotion of the guidelines. This was the first time a parliamentary group had undertaken such a review. The report looked at each of the 12 guidelines and made 136 observations and recommendations on how the British Government could better incorporate each guideline into policy and practice.

In June 2002, a regional workshop was convened in Tobago by the Caribbean Community (CARICOM). Participants from Guyana, Jamaica, Suriname and Trinidad and Tobago explained how their countries' laws and policies measured against the guidelines. The outcome of this workshop was an action plan to support the implementation of priority area one of the Caribbean Regional Strategic Framework on HIV/AIDS, which addresses policy, advocacy and legislation.

National associations—comprising lawyers, other professionals and people living with HIV/AIDS who are united in promoting rights-based approaches to HIV/AIDS — have been formed in many countries. With the support of the United Nations Development Programme, these groups have been encouraged to form regional networks in the regions of Asia and the Pacific, Latin America and the Caribbean and Africa. Other organisations, such as research centres and legal clinics, also promote laws and policies based on human rights. Some also offer legal services to people infected with and affected by HIV/AIDS, who often come from disadvantaged communities and may not possess the information and advocacy skills necessary to participate when laws and policies are debated.

In the common law tradition, international human rights law is persuasive in the interpretation of statutes and the development of national jurisprudence; however, judges and magistrates also need to understand the basic facts about HIV/

AIDS. In September 2001, over 70 judges, magistrates and other lawmakers attended a sensitisation seminar on HIV/AIDS in Lagos, Nigeria, which was hosted by the Centre for the Right to Health.

In 2002, a training package for magistrates who act as Commissioners of Child Welfare was developed in South Africa. The package will help sensitise magistrates to the complex legal and policy issues related to HIV/AIDS that arise in the placement of children in need, many of whom will have been orphaned by AIDS.

Many initiatives that are being undertaken in different contexts and that reflect approaches to law and policy related to HIV/AIDS that have roots in international human rights law. This body of law provides powerful tools for three distinct sectors seeking to address the HIV epidemic.

First, human rights law helps states respond appropriately to the challenges of the HIV/AIDS epidemic by providing a framework on which they can formulate laws and policies that integrate public health objectives and human rights standards.

Second, human rights provide a basis for tools for non-governmental organisations and advocacy groups to use to monitor the performance of states in their policies and programmes and to take action for redress when public health policies violate rights.

Third, human rights also speak to the obligations of public health practitioners with responsibilities for the protection and promotion of health at a population level. In public health itself there is increasing debate about what its ethos and value systems should be in a globalising environment. The emphasis is increasingly on reestablishing a commitment to social justice and popular participation that "locates organised and active communities at the centre as initiators and managers of their own health". For those reasons, public heath practitioners should be familiar with human rights tools and understand their origins, potential and limitations.

REFERENCES

Carrasco E., "Access to Treatment as a Right to Life and Health", *Canadian HIV and AIDS Policy Law Review*; 5: 4, 2000.

Charter of the United Nations (VII), New York: United Nations; 1994; p. 22-8.

Elliott R. Trips and rights: *International human rights law, access to medicines, and the interpretation of the WTO agreement on trade-related aspects of intellectual property rights*, Montreal: Canadian HIV/AIDS Legal Network and AIDS Law Project (South Africa), 2001.

Fidler D.P., *International law and infectious diseases*, New York: Oxford University Press, 1999:210.

International Council of AIDS Service Organisations (ICASO), *An advocate's guide to the international guidelines on HIV/AIDS and human rights*, Toronto: ICASO, 1999.

International Covenant on Economic, Social and Cultural Rights, adopted by General Assembly resolution 2200A (XXI) of 16 December 1966: Article 2(1).

Kirby J., "Human rights and the HIV paradox", *Lancet*, 1996.

Mann JM., Human rights and AIDS: the future of the pandemic. In: Mann J.M., Gruskin S., Grodin M.A., Annas G.J., *Health and human rights*, New York and London: Routledge, 1999:221.

Office of the United Nations Commissioner for Human Rights/ UNAIDS, "HIV/AIDS and Human Rights International Guidelines", Second International Consultation on HIV/AIDS and Human Rights, Geneva, 23–25 September. Geneva: United Nations, 1998.

Second International Consultation on HIV/AIDS and Human Rights (Geneva, 23-25 September 1996). Report of the Secretary-General (E/CN.4/1997/37). Geneva: United Nations, 1997.

UNAIDS, *The UNAIDS guide to the United Nations human rights machinery*, Geneva, 1997.

______________ *Determinants of AIDS-Related Discrimination, Stigmatisation and Denial in India*, Geneva, 2001.

______________, *The UNAIDS guide to the United Nations human rights machinery for AIDS service organisations, people living with HIV/AIDS, and others working in the area of HIV/AIDS and human rights*, Geneva: UNAIDS, 1997

UNAIDS/Inter-ParliamentaryUnion, 1999, *Handbook for legislators on HIV/AIDS, law and human rights: action to combat HIV/*

AIDS in view of its devastating human, economic and social impact, Geneva, 2001.

UNAIDS/WHO (2001), *Sources and prices of selected drugs and diagnostics for people living with HIV/AIDS*, Geneva: UNAIDS (UNAIDS/01.65E).

Universal Declaration of Human Rights, adopted and proclaimed by the United Nations General Assembly Resolution 217 A (III) of 10 December 1948.

United Nations High Commissioner for Human Rights. *The protection of human rights in the context of human immunodeficiency virus (HIV) and acquired immunodeficiency syndrome (AIDS). Commission on Human Rights resolution 1997/33*. Geneva: Office of the United Nations High Commissioner for Human Rights, 1997 (E/CN.4/RES/1997/33).

United Nations General Assembly, *Declaration of commitment on HIV/AIDS*, New York: United Nations, 2001: paragraphs 16, 58 (A/RES/S-26/2).

4

HIV/AIDS: Prevention and Control

Acquired Immune Deficiency Syndrome (AIDS) is a life-threatening condition caused by the Human Immune-deficiency Virus (HIV). Till today, there is no vaccine to protect the community from this dreadful virus. In 1981, researchers have identified two serotypes of HIV. HIV-1 is the predominant serotype worldwide. Eleven subtypes of HIV-1 have been identified. In India, HIV-1 subtype C is the commonest. HIV-2 occurs most commonly in West Africa. Both HIV-1 and HIV-2 cause AIDS and the routes of transmission are the same. However, HIV-2 transmission is slightly less easy and HIV-2 may cause slower progression to AIDS.

Today, HIV is prevalent in all parts of the world and has spread from urban to rural areas, and from individuals practising high risk behaviours to the general population. More and more women attending antenatal clinics are testing HIV-positive, thereby increasing the chances of perinatal transmission.

During sexual intercourse, damage to the lining of sexual organs facilitates transmission of HIV from the infected partner to the uninfected one by exchange of body fluids. It is easier for the virus to be transmitted if the uninfected partner is already suffering from some sexually transmitted disease/ reproductive tract infections, as in this case the lining of the organ is already compromised. The risk of HIV transmission through sharing of needles and syringes by injecting drug users (IDUs), on the other hand is very high. This is because blood is commonly sucked back into the syringe and then re-injected. The risk of HIV from mother to child transmission is believed to be 20-40 per cent in utero, during delivery and after birth. During the post-natal period, transmission of HIV infection from mother to child can occur through breast milk. It is recommended that all HIV mothers should be given an informed choice regarding the advantages and disadvantages of breast-feeding and safer alternatives to breast-feeding.

Prevention is indisputably the most important objective as no curative drug is universally effective and no affordable prevention vaccine is likely to be available in, nor accessible to developing countries in the foreseeable future. Health education and behaviour modification is the prime focus of action for interrupting transmission. It is therefore important to have an information and education programme for all men and women, including adolescents, especially aimed at those who are at greater risk of HIV infection. It is also important to have facilities for detection and treatment of other sexually transmitted infections and to encourage an environment that promotes free and frank dissemination of information without stigmatisation and discrimination against suspected / known cases of HIV/AIDS.

Prevention has maximum impact as part of comprehensive interventions, spearheaded by governments that break the silence around HIV/AIDS and deploy sufficient human and financial resources. Their impact is amplified by wider public health and development strategies addressing the underlying socioeconomic causes that leave people vulnerable to infection, as well as vulnerabilities arising from gender inequities, the denial of human rights and discrimination against marginalised groups. Prevention efforts must be buttressed by well-supported community responses that include people living with HIV/AIDS, religious groups, and traditional and trusted leaders. And, in the context of more effective HIV treatment and the drop in anti-retroviral drug prices, prevention must be linked to the provision of care and support. As the epidemic is constantly shifting, prevention efforts must be tailored to developments in the epidemic, on the research front, and to evaluations that confirm success or failure. Like society itself, the epidemic is in constant flux as it adapts to surrounding factors and circumstances.

The success stories of Cambodia, Senegal, Thailand, Uganda and urban Zambia, as well as those of a number of high-income countries, show that comprehensive prevention approaches are effective. These experiences provide clear evidence of what works:

— *Knowledge is not enough.* Behavioural change requires locally-appropriate, targeted information, training in negotiating and decision-making skills, social and legal support for safer behaviours, access to the means of prevention (e.g., condoms or clean needles) and motivation to change behaviour.

— *The distribution of risk and vulnerability in societies varies greatly, as does the ability to locate and work with specific vulnerable populations.* No single prevention approach can be effective everywhere. To effectively produce and sustain behavioural change on a national scale, focused prevention programmes will involve multiple components, developed with the close input of each targeted population, to address the specific needs of vulnerable groups and the many factors influencing behavioural change.

— *General population efforts are important, especially for the young.* Effective national programmes take into account the need to raise the awareness, knowledge, and HIV prevention and care skills among the rest of the population, especially the young, among whom almost half of all HIV transmission occurs.

— *Partnerships are essential for effective prevention.* Since multiple programmes in multiple populations are needed, it is crucial to create partnerships between different players, including people with HIV/AIDS.

— *Political leadership is essential to an effective response.* Political leadership and action are clearly needed to set the direction for a national response and initiate the development of policies that determine the strategy for managing the epidemic.

— *Half-measures bring, at best, partial results.* Interventions that do not achieve sufficient coverage will simply fail to have a significant impact.

Prevention depends on an environment of openness and inclusion that enables all people, including those living on the margins of society, to undergo voluntary testing, seek and receive treatment, alter their own behaviour, and become allies in the fight against HIV/AIDS. Successful responses challenge stigma and discrimination, protect the rights of those infected and affected by HIV, and include marginalised groups as active participants rather than mere 'beneficiaries' of services.

Prevention efforts have always been hard to implement when access to treatment, care and support is limited. Without the hope of treatment, care and support, and fearing stigma and discrimination, people see little reason to learn about, or disclose, their HIV status. Prevention is enhanced when it is linked to care and support. People are encouraged to come forward and get tested for HIV if they know treatment will be available. For those who test HIV-positive, treatment, care and support not only improve their quality of life, they also decrease the spread of infectious diseases through early diagnosis and treatment. Voluntary counselling and testing services are an entry point for behavioural change; they offer an opportunity for people worried about their serostatus to talk with medical and other trained staff, and discuss how they might prevent further spread of the infection. Open and compassionate care for HIV-infected people helps counter wider societal fears about HIV/AIDS.

Ironically, in some high-income countries where access to treatment and care is widespread, prevention has increasingly become divorced from care. The result has been upturns in risky behaviour and, in some instances, increases in the number of new HIV infections. In such situations, treatment and care efforts must be accompanied by increased and integrated prevention efforts.

EFFECTIVE HIV PREVENTION MEASURES

Effective HIV prevention combines society-wide strategies with particular focus on those parts of the population most at risk. Whatever the extent of the spread of the epidemic, young people need to be at the centre of all HIV strategies—not least because most HIV infections occur during, or soon after, adolescence. Strategies that work combine:

— AIDS life-skills education;
— mass media communication;
— access to condoms;
— voluntary counselling,
— testing and referral;
— treatment of sexually transmitted infections;
— involvement of parents and other adults; and
— efforts to improve young people's social and economic status.

In low-prevalence settings, a concentrated epidemic tends initially to be associated with certain high-risk contexts—typically, sex work, injecting drug users and sex between men. Usually, these activities are also highly stigmatised. But the people at risk in these contexts are not isolated groups; they mix across populations, as confirmed by behavioural surveillance. However, early, large-scale interventions among these groups could stave off a potential epidemic. In high-prevalence settings, the epidemic is spread much more broadly throughout the general population.

The higher the national HIV prevalence rate, the higher the proportion of people who must adopt safer behaviour if the epidemic is to be brought under control. Very high coverage with demonstrably effective interventions then becomes crucial. Whether in low- or high-prevalence areas, the key to effective prevention is to apply essential prevention strategies to the realities of the epidemic, at the local, national or even regional levels.

Twenty years into the HIV/AIDS epidemic, the majority of countries in the world still register national HIV prevalence rates of less than 1 per cent, for the global epidemic is still in its early stages. But two decades ago, there was no country in the world that had nationwide adult HIV prevalence rates above 1 per cent; today there are nearly 50 and, in 12 of them, national adult HIV prevalence is estimated to be more than 10 per cent. HIV rates, reported as a national average, can be misleading. In populous countries, national adult HIV prevalence of, say, 2–3 per cent may nevertheless mean millions of infections. National HIV prevalence rates can also mask the concentrated nature of HIV epidemics in specific parts of the country and among specific populations.

Large-scale epidemics always begin as localised outbreaks before spreading more widely across regions and communities. In Nairobi, Kenya, HIV prevalence among female sex workers surged from 4 per cent in 1981 to 61 per cent in 1985, while prevalence among pregnant women rose from 0 per cent in 1981 to only 2 per cent in 1985, before its subsequent steep rise. The danger signs of impending epidemics are now familiar, but the exact pace of the epidemic's growth still cannot be predicted with certainty. In Thailand, for example, the virus was first detected in 1984, but did not start spreading virulently among sex workers and their clients until five years later. Similarly, in the Nepalese city of Kathmandu, needle-sharing was rife in the early 1990s, yet HIV infections among injecting drug users stayed negligible for six or seven years before rising sharply to the point where, by 1997, nearly half the users were infected.

In Indonesia, anonymous HIV testing of sex workers began in 1988 and, for almost a decade, registered virtually no HIV infection. The results were puzzling because other research was showing that sex work was common, condom use very low, and other sexually transmitted infections highly prevalent. The absence of a HIV epidemic may have been partly because sex workers in Indonesia had a relatively low turnover of partners—around seven in a week, on average, compared with over 30 a week in Thailand at the height of the HIV rise in that country. But new data suggest that there has been a surge in HIV infection among sex workers in some Indonesian locations.

Preventing Sexual Transmission of HIV

The World Health Organisation estimates that over 300 million people are infected each year with curable sexually transmitted infections, a large share of which occur among young people. The presence of such infections magnifies the risk of HIV transmission during unprotected sex as much as tenfold (since the infection creates additional entry points for the virus or facilitates viral replication). Many of these infections (including the four most common: syphilis, gonorrhoea, *chlamydia* and trichomoniasis) can be cured relatively easily with antibiotic treatment. But lack of services, poor availability of drugs, limited access to diagnosis, and disparaging attitudes by service providers are barriers to more effective detection and treatment of sexually transmitted infections as part of HIV/AIDS prevention.

Safe sex is any sexual practice that reduces the risk of transmission of HIV from one person to another. The best protection is by sexual activities that prevent entry of infected semen, vaginal secretions or blood into the mouth, vagina or anus of the partner. These practices include:

i) Staying in a mutually faithful relationship where both partners are uninfected.

ii) Using a condom for all types of sexual intercourse (vaginal, anal or oral) to prevent body secretions containing HIV to come in contact with the skin or mucous membranes of the partner.

iii) Avoiding penetrative sex and replacing it with masturbation, massage, dry kissing and hugging.

iv) Avoiding sex when either partner has open sores or sexually transmitted diseases.

Usage of Condoms

Condoms are the most effective means of protection against the organisms that cause sexually transmitted infection, including HIV. They are effective only if they are used properly during every sexual intercourse. Without access to condoms, many other prevention strategies such as behavioural change communication and sexual and reproductive health education in schools, not to mention family planning campaigns lose much of their potential effectiveness.

The United Nations Population Fund estimates that the number of condoms needed to prevent HIV/ AIDS and other sexually transmitted infections will more than double in the next 15 years. Costs will rise from US$239 million in 2000 to an estimated US$557 million in 2015. This total does not include distribution, training or counselling costs. Low-income countries will need plans that address supply problems along with steady increases in donor support to meet condom costs.

Increasing condom accessibility and availability can increase condom use. In Brazil, there was a massive increase in the uptake of condoms when prices came down in the early 1990s. When Ford South Africa made mass condom distribution part of its HIV/AIDS strategy and put condom distribution machines in workplace toilets, uptake increased 25-fold. However, supply is not the only determinant of condom use. Almost everywhere, sexually active young people are denied information about condoms.

A recent analysis of study samples from eight countries in sub-Saharan Africa found that attitudes towards condom use also depended on the nature of relationships. In marital and regular relationships, many people said that they did not use condoms because they 'trusted' their partner; in regular and casual relationships, people frequently cited a dislike of condoms. This suggests that condom promotion messages need to be tailored to context: couples in steady relationships may need to be convinced that using condoms is a primary means of caring for each other's health.

Condom programming works best as part of a comprehensive 'package' of interventions that include HIV/AIDS education, sexual health and human sexuality, and gender sensitivity training. Since it was first introduced by public health authorities in Ratchaburi Province, Thailand's innovative 100 per cent Condom Use Programme for commercial sex has become known as one of the most effective HIV prevention measures ever.

Preventing HIV Transmission among Homosexuals

In varying degrees, male-to-male HIV transmission is a factor in all HIV epidemics. It has been the predominant mode of transmission of HIV in most high-income countries. In the USA, male-to-male sex accounted for the largest proportion (42 per cent) of annual new infections in 2000, while, in Australia, it accounted for 85 per cent of infections in 2000. Significant HIV prevalence among men who have sex with men has been detected in countries around the world. Where male-to-male sex is repressed legally or through strong social sanctions, men who have sex with men are at especially high risk of HIV infection, since they are harder to identify and reach with preventative services. Countering the discrimination and violence endured by men who have sex with men is therefore a vital part of an effective AIDS response.

Reliable data from countries as diverse as Brazil, Colombia, India, Mexico, Pakistan and Thailand confirm that many men who have unprotected sex with other men also have unprotected sex with women. In Latin America and the Caribbeans, the population of men who have sex with men is diverse, many of the men also have sex with women, HIV rates are significant and, as a result, the epidemic is steadily reaching their female partners. A recent study by the Senegalese National AIDS Commission in Dakar, Senegal, reported that 88 per cent of surveyed men who have sex with men also had sex with women, and 15 per cent were married. Only 14 per cent said they used condoms the last time they had sex. In addition, 37 per cent of the men surveyed reported that they had been raped in the previous year, some by policemen.

Gay communities in high-income countries have been at the forefront of the response to HIV/AIDS, and have mounted very successful prevention efforts, although a resurgence of unsafe sex among men who have sex with men shows the need to constantly renew and reinforce such efforts. In much of Africa and Asia, however, prevention efforts among men who have sex with men have barely begun.

In many middle-and low-income countries, male-to-male sex and HIV transmission tend to be statistically hidden and officially denied. In much of Africa, for example, male-to-male sex is scarcely acknowledged, although self-identified gay groups have been in existence for several years in South Africa and Zimbabwe. Similar groups have recently been formed in Kenya and Senegal.

The Bandhu Social Welfare Society (in Dhaka, Bangladesh) and Sahodaran (in Chennai, India) are community-based agencies providing both outreach and onsite services to men who have sex with men. 'Safe spaces' in their central offices offer stigmatised and marginalised men an opportunity to socialise and to access a range of services. Bandhu Social Welfare Society has an innovative clinic service for sexually transmitted infection diagnosis and treatment and Sahodaran has contributed strongly to national advocacy. Similarly, recent years have seen a series of prevention projects established in

Eastern Europe and Central Asia by gay organisations in collaboration with local authorities, with support from UNAIDS Cosponsors and the UNAIDS Secretariat.

Preventing HIV Transmission among Sex Workers and Their Clients

Sex work is clandestine and illegal in most societies, which makes it difficult to gauge the numbers involved in it. But it is a global phenomenon and a powerful social and economic factor in many countries. By the International Labour Organisation's estimates, the sex work industry accounted for more than 2 per cent of gross domestic product in four South-East Asian countries by the late 1990s. In countries where heterosexual intercourse is the main mode of HIV transmission, HIV epidemics tend to be concentrated initially among sex workers and their clients before becoming established in the wider population. A steep rise in HIV prevalence among sex workers is an alarm signal that HIV rates in the wider population are very likely to increase unless effective prevention efforts are introduced.

Where sex work is widespread but clandestine, this often reflects entrenched gender inequalities. In such places, men's social, economic and political status eclipses that of women, double standards encourage multiple partners for men but not for women, and women's limited educational and livelihood opportunities compel many into some form of sex work. While economic necessity is often the driving motivation for many in sex work, it is not necessarily the only one. Research in the Philippine sex industry, for instance, has found that some sex workers operating out of bars and clubs had worked in formal employment, but opted instead for the slightly lower earnings and risks of the sex trade over the long hours working on assembly lines. Others are coerced into sex work through violence, debt bondage, or trafficking.

It can be difficult or impossible for sex workers to insist on safe sex. Reluctant clients might react with violence or simply move on to someone willing to forego a condom. A recent analysis of condom use by sex workers in Kolkata, India, has found that clients were willing to pay almost double the fee for sex without a condom.

Effective HIV prevention among sex workers addresses the social, economic and legal environments in which they live and work. Sex workers must be involved and empowered through the projects. Efforts must win the cooperation and support of control points in the sex industry, such as brothel owners, bar managers, pimps and the police. It is essential to tackle the prejudice that sex workers endure, and to weave other concerns into the programmes, such as care for their families and children.

When sex work is illegal, it is driven deeper underground, and prevention efforts become more difficult. Sex workers may be subject to police harassment, and carrying condoms can lead to arrest, fines or imprisonment. However, important victories have been won for the protection of sex workers' human rights. Sex workers involved in Bangladesh's Shakti project helped achieve an important court decision recognising sex work as a legal form of income-generation. In Papua New Guinea, the Transex project used a mixture of lobbying and activism to change the attitudes of the local police force, reducing its power over sex workers' lives and preventing it from obstructing the project.

Prevention of HIV Infection via Blood Transfusion

The process of blood collection, transport, storage, testing and distribution, requires maintenance of a certain standard by application of effective quality control mechanism at all levels. Blood is a good medium for growth of any organism because of its nutrient value, adequate oxygen content and optimum temperature. Transfusion of infected blood, therefore, can lead to transmission of blood-borne diseases like hepatitis, syphilis, malaria, and HIV/AIDS. There is an overall acute shortage of blood. The gap between demand and supply of blood is continuously widening due to mushrooming of super-specialist hospitals in urban areas and continuous inappropriate use of blood. It has been estimated that approximately 30 per cent transfusions are either unnecessary or wasteful. Rational and appropriate use of blood and blood products and promotion of voluntary donation can help in overcoming this shortfall.

Blood transfusion should be given only when there is a definite indication to do so and its benefit outweighs the risk associated with it. It is necessary for appropriate use of simple alternatives to transfusion like crystalloids or colloids that are safer and more cost effective. If transfusion cannot be avoided, then specific blood component should be used if possible. Reducing the exposure of patient to different donors will also decrease the risk of transfusion-transmitted diseases. This is of importance in a paediatric patient requiring small quantity of blood every day or on alternate days, who may be transfused with small quantities of blood separated from a single blood unit.

All injections should be avoided as far as possible. Oral medications should be used instead. If injections cannot be avoided, make sure that the needles and syringes are either new disposable ones or appropriately sterilised. Avoid all addictive drugs. If not possible, it is better to use them orally. If injecting drugs cannot be avoided, then the injecting equipment should not be shared. If not possible to avoid sharing equipment, then either boil the equipment for 20 minutes or use fresh bleach solution.

Prevention og HIV Infection among Injecting Drug Users

The illicit drug trade has, over the past 25 years, grown into a multi-billion-dollar industry that spans the planet. By the end of 1999, injecting drug use was being reported in 136 countries; in 114 of them, HIV cases resulting from injecting drug use had been reported. Drug trafficking is now a global phenomenon, touching some 170 countries and territories. It is estimated that up to 10 million people worldwide inject drugs.

Asia is estimated to have the largest number of injecting-drug-related HIV cases. Injecting drug use is also a major factor in HIV epidemics in North America, Western Europe and in parts of Latin America, the Middle East and North Africa. In some Eastern European countries, especially in countries of the former Soviet Union, injecting drug use is driving major HIV/AIDS epidemics among young people, and many outreach programmes report rising numbers of sexually active teenage drug users.

Injecting-drug-related HIV epidemics do not remain limited to injecting drug users. Most injecting drug users are young, male and sexually active. They are likely to acquire or transmit the HIV virus not only by sharing injecting equipment but also through sexual intercourse with regular or casual partners. Injecting drug use also overlaps profoundly with the sex trade, with users often buying sex, or selling sex to finance their drug dependencies. In 2000, in Hanoi, Vietnam, 20 per cent of street-based female sex workers reported recent drug injection, while 23 per cent of male injecting drug users bought sex; in Bangladesh, the corresponding figures were 14 per cent and 50-75 per cent respectively.

Stopping the spread of HIV among injecting drug users requires a comprehensive approach, including drug-dependency treatment and rehabilitation; HIV/AIDS education; access to clean needles/syringes and condoms; legal and social services; and voluntary HIV testing and counselling and psychosocial support. It also requires efforts to deter people (especially young people) from initiating injecting drug use. There is strong evidence to show that effective and humane drug treatment not only reduces drug abuse, but also diminishes HIV risk. A basic ethical principle is that drug control policies must reduce, not augment, the HIV risk faced by drug users, and HIV prevention activities must not inadvertently promote drug abuse.

Small, isolated prevention efforts might slow the pace of the epidemic, but not for long, as Nepal's experience has shown. Needle exchange programmes there began as early as 1991; by

1995, some researchers were claiming that the interventions had averted a HIV epidemic among injecting drug users. But, by 1997, almost half the users tested in Kathmandu were infected with HIV. The needle-exchange programme was too limited and too localised to have a powerful, lasting impact. It had to be expanded. Needle and syringe programmes have also been expanded elsewhere, notably in some countries in Europe and in Australia. In 2000, in England and Wales, there were 420 syringe-distribution programmes, distributing 27 million syringes, equivalent to 180–540 syringes per injecting drug user per year.

Evidence from high- and low-income countries shows that effective prevention and care programmes can be mounted despite the marginalisation, social stigma and legally penalising environment that mark injecting drug users' lives. But the programmes tend to be most successful when laws and police practices facilitate outreach work and service provision to injecting drug users.

For many years, Manipur in India was emblematic of a region in the grip of a rising injecting drug-related HIV epidemic. By the late 1990s, there were already an estimated 40,000 injecting drug users in Manipur, as many as 60 per cent of whom were HIV-positive. To many observers, it seemed a 'lost cause'. But, after studies had revealed that most of the users shared injecting equipment because they feared arrest if caught with needles and syringes, the Society for HIV/AIDS and Lifelines Operations (SHALOM) took the bold step of setting up a needle- and syringe-exchange programme in Churachandpur township. Police were consulted and persuaded not to harass Shalom workers or users found with injecting equipment. HIV incidence among users dropped from almost 77 per cent in 1997 to just under 59 per cent in 2001—still high, but a marked decrease. Persuaded by the effectiveness of the programme, the Manipur Minister of State for Health integrated the approach into the official State AIDS policy.

Bigger official obstacles were cleared in Ukraine, where, in 1998, the parliament added to a HIV/AIDS law the State's guarantee that it would work to facilitate the provision of needle-exchange services for injecting drug users. This hard-won law reform also abolished the mandatory testing of users. Political and public opinion at first had been fearful that the changes would spur drug use and other social problems. But a strong information campaign and widespread public debate gradually convinced voters and legislators that the reforms were ultimately going to benefit all society. Currently, in 2002, 37 needle-exchange projects operate in the country, and are estimated to reach around 20 per cent of all users.

In Brazil, a law was approved by Congress in 2002, authorising the Ministry of Health to establish national policies for specific HIV programmes targeting injecting drug users. A national survey among injecting drug users showed that consistent use of condoms in this population increased from 42 per cent in 1999 to 65 per cent in the year 2000. In the same period, syringe- and needle-sharing decreased from 70 per cent to 41 per cent. As a result, between 1996 and 2000, HIV prevalence among injecting drug users dropped in several cities. In Santos, Sao Paulo State, the drop was from 65 per cent to 42 per cent; in Salvador, from 49 per cent to 7 per cent; and in the city of Rio de Janeiro, from 25 per cent to 8 per cent.

Drug substitution programmes, along with a range of other health and referral services, have been successfully introduced in some places. An example is the Mexican non-governmental organisation, Companeros AC, which has run a programme since the mid-1990s, promoting detoxification and rehabilitation alongside specific HIV-prevention efforts targeting injecting drug users. It helps injecting drug users make behavioural changes that are realistic for them and that are most likely to be sustained—from outright cessation of drug use to adopting less harmful habits.

Fieldwork is carried out in prisons as well as in the wider community. Information leaflets are distributed, along with packages containing condoms, bleach, and education leaflets. Rehabilitation services incorporate complementary treatments such as acupuncture and herbal medicine. Education and support are provided to the families and partners of people who inject drugs.

Prevention of HIV/AIDS from Mother to Child

Prevention of vertical transmission of HIV from mother to child is possible in the following ways:

i) *Antepartum*
   a) Counselling in the antenatal period and HIV testing.
   b) Choice of MTP or continuation of pregnancy.
   c) Correct diet and treatment of anaemia.
   d) Discontinue smoking and illicit drugs.
   e) Regular check up.
   f) Treat RTI/STI.
   g) Detect and treat opportunistic infections.
   h) Antiretroviral therapy.

ii) *Intrapartum*
   a) Delivery in hospital.
   b) Antiretroviral therapy - AZT or Nevirapine.
   c) Do not do amniotomy, foetal scalp blood sampling, foetal scalp electrode monitoring or umbilical blood sampling.
   d) Role of Caesarian Section.

iii) *Postpartum*
   a) Immediate bath to baby.
   b) Breast-feeding vs safer alternatives.
   c) Anti-retroviral therapy to the baby.

HIV infected individuals may suffer from a variety of disorders and develop signs which are suggestive of being infected by

HIV/AIDS. Since sophisticated blood tests may not be available in many developing countries, WHO has laid down clinical criteria for the provisional diagnosis of AIDS. The presence of at least two major signs and one minor sign can be an indication for AIDS provided other causes of depleted immunity are ruled out.

Major signs

i) Weight loss >10 per cent of body weight.

ii) Fever for more than one month, intermittent or continuous.

iii) Chronic diarrhoea for more than one month.

Minor Signs

i) Persistent cough for more than one month.

ii) Generalised dermatitis.

iii) Recurrent herpes zoster.

iv) Oro-pharyngeal candidiasis.

v) Chronic progressive and disseminated herpes simplex infection

vi) Generalised lymphadenopathy.

Counselling and Testing

Counselling and testing has been shown to have a role in both HIV prevention and as an entry point to care. It provides people with an opportunity to learn and accept their HIV status in a confidential environment. This become an integral part of HIV prevention programmes in many countries as it a relatively cost effective intervention in preventing HIV transmission. In India, as HIV testing becomes simpler to perform with the advent of newer kits, the National AIDS Control Organisation has plans for the expansion of testing facilities to all corners of the country in a phased manner.

HIV testing services should be designated to address the multiple needs and rights of individuals at risk or already infected. Such efforts to reduce stigma and discrimination seek to 'normalise' community perceptions of HIV infection and AIDS, and make counselling services available to all who seek them, regardless of their willingness to be tested.

The diagnosis of HIV testing has traditionally been made by detecting antibodies against HIV. There has been rapid evolution in diagnostic technology since the first HIV antibody tests became commercially available. Besides ELISA, newer rapid and simple tests are available which are comparable to ELISA on sensitivity and specificity. In addition they are easy to perform in limited resource settings like district hospitals and more cost-effective than ELISA. The success of counselling and testing strategy largely depends on the availability of cheap testing facilities that give results in the shortest possible time. This makes the rapid tests an attractive option where the client can be subjected to a pretest counselling, test result and post-test counselling in one session.

Counselling should be offered before taking an HIV test. In this process the counsellor prepares the client for the test by explaining what an HIV test is and also by correcting myths and misinformation about HIV/AIDS. This counselling can also be provided to groups to reduce costs and can be backed up by providing printed information. Post-test counselling should always be offered. The idea is to help clients to understand their test results and initiate adaptation to their sero-positive or sero-negative status. When the test is sero-positive, the counsellor tells the client the result clearly and sensitively, providing emotional support and discussing how he/she will cope.

The counsellor must ensure that the person has immediate emotional support from a partner, relative or friend. Sharing one's HIV status with a sexual partner is important to enable the use of safer sexual practices and should be encouraged. Counselling is also important when the test result is negative. While the client is likely to feel relief, the counsellor needs to discuss changes in behaviour that can help the client to stay negative.

HIV/AIDS is a disease with long incubation period. People suffering from this condition require long-term, continuous treatment. Hospital care in such conditions is not feasible. So, home-based care is absolutely necessary for such cases. Home-based care has some specific objectives:

i) Formation of indispensable teams, which will train the family members who will provide social support and teach prevention. They will develop referral network linking health services with NGOs.
ii) *Clinical management:* A proper diagnosis and treatment.

About two decades have passed since HIV/AIDS has entered the medical horizon. As yet, no curative treatment has been found. However, four years after the virus was discovered, the first drug for treatment of HIV infection was discovered. Scientists discovered agents that act on the life cycle of the virus in the body and stop viral replication.

The first drug, which was discovered in 1987, acted on the reverse transcriptase enzyme to prevent formation of pro- virus DNA. Since then, various drugs acting on reverse transcriptase have been discovered. Two groups of drugs:

i) Nucleoside Analogues and
ii) Non-nucleoside analogues were discovered till 1998.

In 1998, another group of drugs called protease inhibitors was discovered and announced in the World Congress of AIDS in Vancouver. These were the drugs, which acted on the enzyme protease, which helped in the maturation of m-RNA to mature virions. All these anti retroviral drugs act on various stages of the life cycle of the virus in the human body and stop the replication of the virus but do not eradicate the virus out of the human cell where they are firmly integrated.

NEW PREVENTION TECHNOLOGIES

Potential technologies currently being pursued also hold the promise of radically changing the landscape of HIV/AIDS prevention. The most prominent are microbicides and vaccines against HIV.

Microbicides

As a form of 'chemical condom' that can be self-administered, microbicides could increase the options for women and men who find it difficult or impossible to persuade their partners to use a condom. Acceptability studies in South Africa, Uganda and Zimbabwe suggest that women who seldom or never use condoms could reduce their overall risk of infection if an effective microbicide were available to them at low cost.

Applied inside the vagina or rectum, a microbicide is intended to prevent infection with HIV and, possibly, other bacterial and viral sexually transmitted infections. It can be produced as a gel, cream, suppository, sponge or in other forms, and may also have contraceptive (spermicidal) properties. The ideal product would be odourless and colourless, and therefore undetectable to partners who refuse other forms of protection.

After the disappointment of the Phase III trial of nonoxynol-9 gel, an estimated 56 new products are in various stages of development, from pre-clinical stages to Phase III effectiveness trials. While no major pharmaceutical company has thus far invested in the development of a microbicide, research into this preventive option has recently been spurred by several grants from the Bill and Melinda Gates Foundation. The International Working Group on Microbicides, which includes public agencies from around the world among its members, continues to promote and facilitate the development of microbicides.

Vaccines

Research to find a vaccine against HIV has been making steady progress in the past 10 years. Unfortunately, 'steady' is not fast enough for all the people who could benefit from it. Even if current attempts to speed up the research process and programmes for the introduction of vaccines are successful, there is little chance that vaccination against HIV will be available on a large scale before the end of the decade.

An estimated US$400–500 million is currently spent on HIV vaccine research annually, with most of this going into basic research. Institutions involved in the global HIV vaccine effort include the US National Institutes of Health, the International AIDS Vaccine Initiative (IAVI), the US Centers for Disease Control and Prevention, the French *Agence Nationale de Recherches sur le SIDA* (ANRS), the European Community (through the EUROVAC programme), and several biotechnology and pharmaceutical companies. National AIDS vaccine research programmes are ongoing in Australia, Canada, Japan, Sweden, the United Kingdom and the United States of America. Low- and middle-income countries (including Brazil, China, Cuba, Haiti, India, Kenya, South Africa, Thailand, Trinidad and Tobago, and Uganda) are also actively involved in vaccine development and trials. WHO and UNAIDS have been actively supporting these national AIDS vaccine programmes.

Despite all this activity, the peculiarities of the HIV virus make finding a vaccine difficult and expensive. HIV differs from most other infectious diseases in that the virus directly attacks white blood cells that are central to directing the body's immune responses, leaving them incapable of controlling infection or preventing disease. 'Classical' vaccines, based on an entire microorganism (viruses or bacteria) that has been killed or rendered harmless, may not be safe enough to use against HIV as they could lead to HIV infection.

Experimental HIV vaccines are therefore primarily based on parts of the virus, which makes the development of a vaccine even more challenging. The multiple variants of HIV pose a further complication. Ten subtypes of the HIV-1 virus have been identified, and are distributed in different parts of the world. Researchers do not yet know whether a broadly protective vaccine will be possible or if a separate vaccine will be needed for each subtype.

The most prevalent HIV subtypes are A and C, present in different regions in Africa, but the majority of the vaccines currently in trials are modelled on the genetic profile of subtype B—the one predominant in high-income countries. Finally, HIV vaccine research remains a 'highrisk/ low-return investment' for private sector industry. This is only partly because the greatest need for the vaccine is among low-income countries. An even greater obstacle—at least currently—is the inadequate scientific understanding of the mechanisms by which the virus evades the body's natural immune responses. Consequently, it is not known exactly what immune responses are necessary to prevent or control HIV infection.

Developing a HIV vaccine is an arduous process. Experimental vaccines are first tested on animals, and the best vaccine candidates are then selected for possible testing on humans. Testing is then carried out on healthy volunteers in three phases.

Phase I trials are done on 20–40 volunteers to confirm the vaccine's safety and whether it triggers useful HIV-specific immune responses.

Phase II tests involve hundreds of volunteers to further check safety and assess the potency of immune responses.

Phase III tests can last up to four years and involve field trials with thousands of volunteers, some of whom receive the vaccine while others form a control group.

Extremely complicated from the logistical, scientific and ethical points of view, these trials assess whether the candidate vaccine protects against HIV infection or the onset of AIDS. Definitive results of the first Phase III trials of a candidate vaccine based on gp120 (an external protein of HIV) are expected in 2003.

The first Phase III trial, with 5400 volunteers, has been ongoing in the United States, Canada and the Netherlands since 1998, and is based on subtype B. The second Phase III trial began in 1999 in Thailand, and is based on the B and E subtypes prevalent there, involving 2500 volunteers. Planning is under way to initiate a Phase III trial of another approach in Thailand in 2003, and additional candidate vaccines are entering Phase I/II trials.

An African AIDS Vaccine Programme, announced in Nairobi in June 2000, is bringing together African scientists, governments and institutions. They aim to complete at least one efficacy trial by 2007.

While a useable vaccine is still many years away, discussion has begun on how to implement vaccination programmes once one exists. Usually, vaccines only arrive in low-and middle-income countries many years after they have recouped their costs in high-income countries. This cannot be allowed to occur with effective HIV vaccines, which need to be rapidly available and affordable to all who need them.

Mechanisms to ensure simultaneous access to AIDS vaccines in both low- and high-income countries must be prepared long before a vaccine is developed, in order to provide quick access to those who need it. The International AIDS Vaccine Initiative and others are proposing significant changes to existing approaches to vaccine production, licensing, pricing, purchasing and distribution. Among other issues is the need to harmonise national regulations and international guidelines governing vaccine approval and use.

An important technical challenge will be that of creating the necessary production capacity, and supporting it with reliable estimates of demand for specific vaccines. Many of the challenges in ensuring that a vaccine is available—and affordable—are similar to those relating to expanding access to antiretroviral drugs.

Differential pricing, together with financial support from donors, will almost certainly be necessary for low-income countries. Technical assistance and coordination by international agencies will be needed. There are policy conundrums, too. Since the vaccination will not immediately be available to everyone, costs and benefits have to be calculated to determine where the initial focus should be. Policymakers must also decide what to do if the first available vaccines are only marginally effective or have significant side effects.

WHO, UNAIDS and IAVI have collaborated on a study aimed at estimating the need for, and probable uptake of, preventative vaccines based on two potential scenarios: a low/ moderate-efficacy vaccine (30–50 per cent effective) and a high-efficacy vaccine (80–90 per cent effective). A vaccination programme using a low/ moderate-efficacy vaccine would need to be accompanied by intensive positive-behaviour counselling, so as not to undermine existing prevention efforts. Furthermore, it would be likely to have the most benefit if vaccination were targeted at populations most vulnerable to HIV infection. A high-efficacy vaccine could be delivered to larger segments of the general population. Although it is difficult to predict the uptake of vaccines, in the absence of information on the cost of the vaccine itself and on the requirements for delivery, the study concluded that the probable uptake would be far less than the estimated need, both for a low/moderate- and a high-efficacy vaccine.

The unique stigma associated with HIV/AIDS may significantly hinder the uptake of HIV vaccination, once it becomes available. Discrimination faced by many of the communities most vulnerable to HIV infection may prevent individuals from coming forward for vaccination, particularly if programmes are focused only at individuals who might be at high risk of infection. When an effective HIV vaccine is available, the international community and affected countries will have to make many critical decisions on how to use it. Extra investment in HIV/AIDS prevention and control will be necessary.

REFERENCES

Alexander P., "Contextual risk versus behaviour: The impact of the legal, social and economic context of sex work on individual risk taking", *Research for Sex Work*; 4, Amsterdam, 2001

Burrows D, Landman W., "Harm reduction: A key component of fighting AIDS in Russia", *Sexual Health Exchange* 2001-2; p. 5–7., 2002.

Centers for Disease Control and Prevention, *Need for Sustained HIV Prevention for Gay and Bisexual Men: HIV Infections Continue at High Levels among Men of All Races with Dramatic Impact among Men of Color*, Atlanta: National Center for HIV, STD and TB Prevention, 2000.

_______________ *HIV/AIDS Update—A glance at the HIV epidemic*, Atlanta: Centers for Disease Control and Prevention (CDC), 2001.

Crofts N., et al., "Harm Reduction in Asia: A successful response to hidden epidemics", *AIDS*; 12 (supplement B): S109–S115, 1998.

Delor F, Hubert M., "Revisiting the concept of 'vulnerability'", *Social Science & Medicine*; 50: 1557–1570, 2000.

Grosskurth H et al.. "Control of sexually transmitted diseases for HIV prevention: understanding the implications of the Mwanza and Rakai trials", *The Lancet*, 2000.

UNAIDS, "Innovative approaches to HIV prevention", *Best Practice Collection*, Geneva, 2000.

_______________ , *Accelerating Access to HIV/AIDS Care, Treatment and Support*, Geneva, 2001.

_______________ *Reaching out, scaling up: eight case studies of home and community care for and by people with HIV/AIDS*, Geneva, 2001.

_______________ ,WHO, *Key elements in HIV/AIDS care and support*, Geneva, 2000.

UNDP, "HIV/AIDS: *Implications for Poverty Reduction*, New York, 2001.

_______________ , *Strategic resource guide: strategies for action to combat HIV/AIDS within the education sector*, Ghana, 2001.

_______________ , *UNESCO's strategy for HIV/AIDS preventive education*, Paris, 2001.

World Bank, *Confronting AIDS: public priorities in a global epidemic*, Oxford: Oxford University Press for the World Bank, 1999.

5

Prevention of Mother-to-Child Transmission of HIV

Mother-to-Child Transmission (MTCT) is by far the commonest and most important route of transmission for newborns and infants, and it accounts for more than 95 per cent of childhood infections in SSA. By the end of 2001, UNAIDS estimated that 2.7 million children (<15 years) were living with HIV/AIDS, most of them in SSA. In 2002 alone, it was estimated that 800,000 children were infected with HIV.

HIV is reversing gains in child survival and development and impacting negatively on mortality rates of children under age five among the most affected countries in SSA. In 2000, the number of women infected with HIV equalled that of men for the first time. As the number of HIV-infected women of child-bearing age increases, the number of HIV-infected infants (and orphans) is also expected to increase.

An HIV-infected pregnant woman can infect her baby during pregnancy (in utero), during labour and delivery (peripartum), or after birth through breast-feeding (postnatal). The risk of infection is now thought to be 5-10 per cent during pregnancy, 10-20 per cent during labour and delivery, and 5-20 per cent during breast-feeding. Regardless of when transmission occurs, the greatest single determinant of mother-to-child transmission of HIV is maternal viral load; the higher it is, the higher the risk of transmission.

Table 1
Range of transmission rates of HIV from mother-to-child

Period	*Transmission rate*
During pregnancy	5-10 per cent
During labour and delivery	10-20 per cent
During breast-feeding	5-20 per cent
Overall without breast-feeding	15-30 per cent
Overall with breast-feeding until 6 months	25-35 per cent
Overall with breast-feeding until 18 to 24 months	30-45 per cent

HIV transmission during Pregnancy: The placenta is an organ lining the uterus (womb) of a pregnant woman, providing food for the developing baby through the umbilical cord. The placenta also provides an efficient barrier against many infectious agents. HIV transmission risk increases if:

— The mother has a viral, bacterial, or parasitic placental infection during pregnancy impairing the placental protective function.

— The mother acquires her initial HIV infection during the pregnancy and, therefore, develops a very high viral load for a short time, before she has time to build an immune response.

— The mother has severe immune deficiency associated with AIDS.

HIV transmission during labour and delivery: Infants have the greatest chance of becoming infected with HIV during labour and delivery. Infection is facilitated by:

— Exposure to blood and secretions that contain HIV in the birth canal through the infants' mucous membranes, or through disruption of their skin.

— Placental separation with mixing of maternal/foetal blood.

— Instrumentation or scalp monitoring, which may provide an entry site for HIV. Prolonged rupture of membranes leading to a longer duration of exposure to maternal secretions.

— Swallowing HIV in maternal blood or secretions resulting in exposure through the gastrointestinal tract.

— Prolonged time to negotiate the birth canal.

HIV transmission during breast-feeding: We know that HIV is present in breast milk. Transmission risk increases with:

— Mixed feeding (giving both breast and artificial feeds). Exposure to any food other than breast milk may increase the risk of contamination and hence inflammation of the intestinal tract in those babies who breast-feed.

— Maternal mastitis or cracked nipples.

— Sores in the baby's mouth.

— Prolonged duration of breast-feeding.

— Maternal vitamin A deficiency

A COMPREHENSIVE APPROACH TO PREVENTION OF MOTHER-TO-CHILD TRANSMISSION

The World Health Organisation (WHO) has proposed a four-pronged approach to Prevention of Mother-to-Child Transmission (PMTCT). The details are given in Table 2.

Table 2

A framework for action to prevent HIV infection in infants and young children

All women prevent	→	HIV infection
HIV-infected women	→	prevent unintended pregnancy
HIV-infected pregnant	→	women prevent MTCT
HIV-infected women, their infant and family	→	provide care and support

Preventing HIV infection in women will significantly contribute to PMTCT. Family planning services need to be expanded so that all women, whether HIV-positive or -negative, may receive care and support to prevent or delay future pregnancies. Many women in developing countries are unaware of their serostatus.

Four specific interventions to reduce mother-to-child transmission of HIV are integrated into MCH clinics:

i) Voluntary testing and counselling (VTC)
ii) Enhanced obstetric care and adoption of safer obstetric practices for all women
iii) Antiretroviral use (NVP)
iv) Infant feeding counselling, and ongoing support and follow-up for HIV-positive women.

The WHO endorses this as part of the minimum package of care for all pregnant women. Even as efforts continue to prevent HIV infection, many women and their families are already infected with HIV, and even with the best efforts to prevent MTCT, some infants will still get infected. Providing care and support to HIV-infected women, their infants, and their families is a moral imperative, and it gives credibility to continuing prevention efforts. Midwives, physicians, nurses, or other trained health care workers are the usual providers of PMTCT services, including VTC, safer obstetric practices, treatment with NVP, and infant feeding counselling, all of which are integrated into antenatal, obstetric, neonatal, and postpartum care.

The goals of the PMTCT programme are to:

— Reduce the risk of transmission of HIV and other STIs from mother to child.
— Integrate PMTCT into routine prenatal care.
— Train health workers in maternity settings in PMTCT principles and counselling.

— Dispel myths and provide accurate information on HIV to mothers, their children, their families, and their communities.
— Promote both the primary and secondary prevention of HIV.
— Encourage care and support of HIV-infected and affected persons, including orphans. Promote mutual support, self-esteem, and self-determination among HIV-infected mothers and their families via support groups and microenterprise loans.

VOLUNTARY TESTING AND COUNSELLING

In a PMTCT programme, four types of counselling performed: HIV pre- and post-test counselling, infant feeding counselling, and ongoing counselling. Ongoing counselling includes:

— Reinforcement of infant feeding counselling and support
— Support to disclose to partners and significant others
— FP information and services to delay or prevent unintended pregnancies
— Support to adopt "positive living"
— Encouragement to join a mothers' support group
— Support during infants' testing and diagnosis
— Psychological and spiritual support

As in other areas of counselling, the PMTCT counsellor's roles are to listen to an individual's concerns, to ask questions, and to provide information and emotional support. Counselling is not the same as giving advice or telling people what they should do.

Prenatal Interactive Group Discussions

The purpose of group discussions is to talk about important facts related to pregnancy and HIV. It is also used to prepare the client for the later events of testing and post-test counselling.

The group discussions reduce the long waiting period. They are also a major step in creating rapport and providing accurate and standardised information which women can discuss amongst themselves during and after the group session. The group discussion takes advantage of the familiar health education sessions, but also enhances these more traditional approaches with information pertinent to HIV, nutrition, and pregnancy. A PMTCT service provider who is trained in the basic principles, skills, and approach to PMTCT facilitates the discussions. Messages at this stage are tailored for women whose HIV status is unknown. The messages communicate the advantages of HIV testing and the opportunity to have testing done.

The counsellor should follow the following steps in the prenatal group discussion:

— Introduce yourself and clarify your role.

— Use simple language that can be understood by your audience.

— Take note of your appearance and dress, because dress and posture can affect the message.

— Take note of body movement, language, and techniques that may affect your audience.

— Encourage your audience to participate through engaging them to make comments and ask questions during the session.

— Make it lively and humorous.

— Common questions asked by participants include benefits of PMTCT services for the mother, how best to motivate partners to come to ANC clinics, and how best to approach disclosure of HIV test results to partners.

What to Say

— Find out why the clients have come for prenatal care-ask questions.

— Let the clients know that their health and their babies' health are our concern.

— Let the clients know that a variety of laboratory tests, including urinalysis, haemoglobin, syphilis tests, and blood grouping, are commonly performed to optimise prenatal care.

— Explain the first four tests. In particular, explain the nature of syphilis, and explain that it can be transmitted from mother to infant if the mother (and father) are not appropriately treated. Ask the clients if they know of any "new" disease that can similarly affect a mother and her infant. Most often that answer will be HIV/AIDS.

— Affirm that HIV can indeed be transmitted from mother to child, and take the opportunity to review the basic facts about HIV/AIDS.

— Talk about modes of HIV transmission. MTCT is not generally a well-known mode of transmission and you need to explain it well. Emphasise that not all infants of HIV-infected mothers acquire the infection.

Explain the difference between HIV and AIDS.

— Explain that an HIV test provides the mother and the health care provider with opportunities to reduce the risk of MTCT. Mention that NVP reduces viral load and reduces chances of infection during labour and delivery by 50 per cent.

— Mention that the HIV test is free at this point in time but it may not always be.

— Inform them that they will have an opportunity for a subsequent discussion with a counsellor in private. Emphasise that if they choose to take an HIV test, their results will be kept confidential.

— Mention that, though their results will be kept confidential, it is in their interest to share their results with partners and other significant persons (including health care providers) who may be in a position to provide care and support.

— Find out how the clients plan to share their results with their partner(s) and advise them to avoid discussing the results in anger. The issue should be discussed at an appropriate time and place.

— Encourage the clients to come to clinic with their partners.

— Find out whether the clients remember what tests need to be done.

— Direct clients where to go for their individual session with the counsellor.

— Emphasise that exclusive breast-feeding for at least six months is the optimal way for women in developing countries to feed their infants. The specifics of infant feeding options are best discussed later with individual women, based on knowledge of their HIV status and their specific circumstances.

What Not to Do

— Do not ask who is willing to do the test in a group setting. Consent is given in private and on an individual basis.

— void judgmental statements.

Individual Pretest Consent

The purpose of individual consent is to provide the clients private time with the counsellor in order to ask questions and seek clarification. All first visit ANC clients should receive information and counselling about HIV and MTCT. Interact with the client in a clear, respectful, and non-judgmental dialogue, with more listening than instructing.

The counsellor should:

— Introduce yourself, and again emphasise the confidential nature of HIV VTC and related services.

— Ask about the current pregnancy.

— Find out whether the client can still recall the tests to be done in order to be sure that she is informed. Ask specifically if she recalls what was discussed about HIV and HIV testing. Ask her if there are any of the prenatal lab tests, including the HIV test, which she does not want.

- Remind her that her results will be given back on the same day. For mothers who refuse an HIV test, accept their decision and assure them that it will not be done without their consent, even though blood is drawn for other antenatal tests. Let them know that the test can be done at a future visit, if they change their minds. Reassure mothers who refuse an HIV test that it will not in any way affect the quality of their future care.
- Inform mothers that you are going to ask them a few questions that will help you to understand what needs to be done to prevent HIV. Ask the questions in a simple way so that the client can understand and respond to them.
- Remember, the questions are sensitive, so do not reveal your reactions to the answers.
- Neatly record all information in the register, and ensure that the consent form is signed.
- Circle on the lab slip all the tests to which the patient consents.
- Make sure the correct ID is written to avoid confusion in the lab.
- Tell the client where to go after the specimen has been collected.
- Let her know that she will see you later for post-test counselling.

Post-Test Counselling

Post-test counselling helps the client decide what to do and how to deal with her feelings in relation to the test results. Post-test counselling is necessary for all the clients irrespective of their test results.

The counsellor should:

- Use his/her judgement or observation to determine how the client is feeling when she comes for her results.
- Take note that every human being fears the unknown.
- Assess the client's ability to cope with bad news and the availability of psychological and spiritual support within her own family and cultural context.
- Be sensitive to the patient's feelings of vulnerability, anxiety, and fear, and treat her the way you yourself would like to be treated if you were in her shoes. Always allow the client time to react to her HIV results.
- Ask if she understands what her results mean, and explain again what they mean.

If the results are negative

- Tell the client that you have her test results, and ask her if she is ready for them.
- Tell the client her results clearly, e.g., "Your test result shows that you are HIV-negative."
- Allow the client time to react to her HIV results.
- Explain what an HIV-negative test result means.
- Remind the client of the possibility of a window period and advise her to repeat the test in three to six months, while avoiding exposure to HIV in the interim. This next test is an opportunity for her to undertake HIV testing with her partner.
- Ask the client what she will do to remain negative and encourage her. Explain the importance of Abstinence/Be faithful/Condom use.
- Give HIV/AIDS brochures to the client, and encourage her to show them to her partner.
- Write "Post-test counselling done (PTCD)—HIV negative" in consultation and ANC cards.

If the results are positive

— Assess her ability to cope with bad news and the availability of psychological and spiritual support within her own family and cultural context.

— Consider asking, "If one of your friends was infected with HIV, what would you advise them?" Much of the post-test counselling can then be done as a hypothetical situation, before actual disclosure of the HIV test result. After learning of the positive test result, the woman may not remember much of the counselling.

— Ensure that she is ready to receive the test result before you disclose it. Use sensitive and inoffensive language and terminology that is easily understood by the patient.

— Differentiate between being HIV-infected and having AIDS. HIV-infected persons usually remain healthy. AIDS may not develop for many years (average 10 years after infection).

— Discuss risk reduction strategies including ways to avoid sexual transmission of HIV to a partner(s).

— Explain the importance of abstinence/be faithful/condom use. Abstinence and "safer sex" are two possible options. Talk about partner testing and mutual monogamy.

— Tell her what to do in order to maintain or improve her health (i.e., abstain from sexual intercourse if possible, or use condoms consistently and correctly if abstinence is not possible, avoid alcohol and tobacco, eat a well-balanced diet, seek prompt treatment for sexually transmitted infections and opportunistic infections, and maintain good personal and environmental hygiene).

— Talk about future pregnancy and child bearing—the effect of pregnancy on HIV, the effect of HIV on pregnancy, and the risk for the infant. Discuss family planning options: condom use plus a second method, including postpartum tubal ligation, if available.

— Describe HIV+ support group activities, if available, and recommend enrolment in a support group.

— Discuss NVP treatment for herself and her baby. Each site should decide whether to give it at 34-36 weeks gestation or to give it at the first ANC visit. All HIV-positive pregnant women should have NVP (200 mg) available to self-administer when they begin labour.

— Find out if she understands this advice.

— Briefly discuss infant feeding. Give her time to think about it for further discussion at the next visit (this may not be appropriate for a woman with an advanced pregnancy). Discuss partner notification technique. Offer to counsel the spouse/partner, either together with the patient or privately.

— Give HIV/AIDS brochures to the client and encourage her to show them to her partner. Write "Post-test counselling done or (PTCD)—Administer NVP (200 mg) in labour" in consultation and ANC cards.

— Obtain permission to make follow-up visits, if the patient (or her baby) does not return for her scheduled prenatal, postpartum, or infant welfare visits.

— Praying with the patient is often helpful. If you pray with her, be sensitive to and respectful of her own religious beliefs. Be compassionate, not judgmental. She will need your ongoing support later, in follow-up counselling sessions, after the initial shock is over.

— Balance information provided with the mother's state of mind—consider postponing some of the discussions until the next visit.

Post-Delivery Counselling of HIV-Infected Mothers

— Check on the OB ward of participating health facilities every day to arrange appropriate follow-up for HIV-positive mothers and their babies and ensure they have been treated with NVP.

— Accurately record all information on the PMTCT follow-up register. Duration of ruptured membranes and time of administration of maternal and infant NVP doses relative to time of delivery are important, because they greatly influence MTCT rates.

— Educate the mother (and/or other family members who will participate in raising the child) in the following: safe preparation of formula vs exclusive breast-feeding for six months; infection risk-reduction practices; nutrition for mother and baby; principles of routine well baby care and immunisations; need for early identification and treatment of opportunistic infections (OIs); and importance of infant follow-up for PCR and HIV antibody testing.

— Review the ABCs of HIV prevention and "safer sex". Review family planning options. If patient desires a postpartum tubal ligation, make necessary arrangements and obtain consent for surgery and sterilisation.

— Help the mother reaffirm her decision about the method of infant feeding she will use and help her initiate that method.

— Check the health status of the baby and mother. This may require clinical and laboratory evaluation of their HIV disease staging, in addition to routing postpartum care.

— Encourage mothers with active TB or mothers who look too sick to breast-feed to feed their babies with infant formula rather than breast milk. Find out if there is someone in the family who can be trained to prepare the formula, and discuss the implications of disclosure with the mother.

— Explain the importance of follow-up. Arrange follow-up appointments for mother and baby.

— Provide family planning information, counselling, and methods appropriate for both breast-feeding and non-breast-feeding mothers.

— Give the client a lab slip stating when she should come back with the infant for immunisation and PCR collection.

Find out the specific address of the client and seek permission to visit her at home. Reassure her that, during such a visit, you would respect confidentiality.

— Emphasise your availability for further information, counselling, and support whenever she needs it, including facilitating disclosure to the partner and offering VTC.

Confidentiality

Confidentiality can be defined as maintaining privacy or secrecy of communication; not telling anyone else what you know about someone; keeping secret that knowledge with which the patient has entrusted you. The only exception is health care providers sharing information with one another so they can provide optimal care for HIV-infected patients. An example is midwives, counsellors, nutritionists, and others who participate in the care of an HIV-positive mother in the context of PMTCT. They need to know her status in order to provide appropriate services. On the other hand, the laboratory staff not directly involved in her testing and the records clerk do not need to know her results and therefore should not be told.

Confidentially is an aspect of the ethical code, which is vital in all professions, especially in the health care profession, and particularly in the setting of HIV/AIDS. It helps establish trust between the client and counsellor. It increases uptake of VTC, reduces worry to the individual and maintains dignity. The client feels respected and is therefore likely to come back to continue receiving care. It gives the client a sense of control and autonomy over her life, even with an illness such as HIV/AIDS. To enable the client to achieve confidentiality:

— Counsel in a quiet place that is free from visitors.

— Record results in such a way that only health care workers (HCWs) can understand.

— Store results and other confidential records in a place that is accessible only to HCWs who care for the patient.

— Maintain confidentiality regardless of whether a client is negative or positive. It may seem harmless, even complimentary, to talk about a client's negative HIV results.

— The patient may share her results with a group of trusted family members and friends who maintain "shared confidentiality." However, sharing this information is the patient's prerogative. The counsellor's role is to support the client, whether she chooses to share or not to share her results.

— Avoid VTC procedures that may inadvertently identify women as being HIV-positive.

— Seek the client's consent to visit her at home, if home visits are feasible. When PMTCT staff visit, they must keep discussions private, unless otherwise indicated by the client. When initiating HIV-positive mothers' support groups, seek mothers' permission prior to scheduling a meeting of positive mothers.

NEVIRAPINE TREATMENT

Nevirapine (NVP) (generic name) or Viramune (trade name) is a non-nucleoside reverse transcriptase inhibitor (NNRTI) used in combination with other anti-retroviral drugs to treat HIV/AIDS. It works by lowering the viral load and allowing the body's immunity to recover, especially when it is taken in combination with other drugs. Boehringer-Ingelheim (BI) Pharmaceutical Company makes NVP in 200 mg tablets and as a liquid suspension of 50 mg in 5 ml, and donates the drug for use in PMTCT programmes.

Dosage and Administration

Maternal dose:: Guidelines for the caretaker

i) For PMTCT of HIV, the HIV-infected pregnant mother should swallow one 200 mg dose orally as soon as active labour begins. Studies have shown that higher cord blood levels of NVP are found when HIV-positive women self-administer the drug at the onset of labour, instead of waiting until they arrive at a health care facility, suggesting that self-administration of NVP by women at the onset of labour is more efficacious.

ii) Dispense one wrapped 200 mg tablet of NVP with written instructions to all HIV-infected pregnant women at the first ANC visit or at 34-36 weeks of pregnancy to take home and keep safely until the onset of labour. No studies have been reported on optimal timing of dispensation of NVP to the mothers (first ANC vs 34-36 weeks). CBCHB is currently evaluating which time results in the highest treatment rates. At each ANC visit, ask if the woman still has the NVP and reinforce instructions to swallow the NVP tablet at the onset of labour, to record the date and time on the instruction sheet, and to go immediately to the facility where she will deliver.

iii) For any woman who has lost the NVP, dispense another dose. Instruct her that, if she goes into labour and delivers in a facility without a PMTCT programme, she should still take her tablet at the onset of labour as directed. She should bring her baby to a participating facility as soon as possible after delivery, to get NVP for the infant. The baby should ideally receive the NVP at 48-72 hours after birth.

iv) When the woman arrives at the labour ward, check the prenatal record for the order, "Administer NVP in labour," which indicates that the HIV test was positive and that the woman is participating in the NVP Programme. Record whether or not she took her NVP tablet before arrival. If she took it before arrival, record on the medical record and on the follow-up register the date and time she took it. If she did not take her NVP before arrival, record on the maternity register the date and time you gave her the tablet on the maternity ward.

v) For patients who did not receive NVP in ANC or who state they lost the tablet, verify the mother's status and give her NVP (200 mg) as soon as you are sure she is in true labour.

vi) If the mother delivers less than two hours after receiving NVP, there will not have been enough time for the drug to cross the placenta to achieve an adequate blood level in the baby's body. Treat the baby as outlined in #5 under "B: Infant Dose."

vii) When the HIV status of a woman in early labour is not known, offer VTC. If she consents to testing and NVP prophylaxis, perform the test as soon as possible and, if positive, administer NVP during labour.

viii) If a woman who has never had VTC arrives in advanced labour (delivery imminent in <2 hours), postpone VTC until shortly after delivery. If she accepts testing, perform test as soon as possible so that, if she is infected, you can treat the newborn as in number 5 under "B: Infant Dose."

ix) If >48 hours has elapsed since the woman took NVP, repeat the 200 mg dose when labour is progressing well.

x) For women who do not consent to VTC, each PMTCT programme will have to decide whether or not to administer NVP. The CBCHB PMTCT programme does not administer NVP to women who refuse testing because the acceptance rate is over 90 per cent.

xi) If the woman vomits within 30 minutes of taking the NVP, repeat the dose as soon as she is stable.

xii) For breast-feeding HIV-positive mothers who did not receive NVP prior to delivery, there is currently insufficient evidence for or against giving NVP postpartum to reduce breast milk transmission during the newborn period, when the baby is most susceptible to acquiring HIV from breast milk. Until studies are done to determine whether postpartum maternal NVP reduces breast milk transmission, each facility will need to decide whether or not to treat those mothers postpartum with NVP.

Infant dose

i) Give the baby's dose of 2 mg/kg body weight at 48-72 hours after birth.

ii) If the baby is to be discharged before 48 hours, give the dose just prior to discharge.

iii) If you are unable to weigh the baby, administer a fixed 0.6 ml dose, as this approximates the recommended dose for a newborn of average weight.

iv) Although 48-72 hours is ideal, the infant's NVP dose can be given up to seven days postpartum, if the infant is brought in late for any reason.

v) If an HIV-positive mother delivers before receiving NVP, give the baby an initial dose of NVP as soon as possible after birth; then give a second dose to baby after 48-72 hours or just prior to discharge, if discharged before 48 hours.

vi) If the baby vomits within 30 minutes of taking NVP, repeat the dose as soon as the patient is stable.

Subsequent Pregnancies

If women who have had PMTCT interventions subsequently return with another pregnancy, it is not necessary to test them again, unless they question their positive test result. Provide support and counselling again about MTCT, use of NVP, and infant feeding options. Inquire as to whether this was a planned pregnancy. Find out her thoughts about future pregnancies. Offer FP information and counselling during ANC, especially if she plans to delay or avoid further pregnancy. The most common reason given for subsequent unintended pregnancy is failure to disclose to partners. Therefore, mothers require support in this area.

Side Effects

These include allergic reaction, nausea, fatigue, diarrhoea, fever, vomiting, and hepatitis.

Preparation for Infant NVP Administration

NVP is available as a ready-to-use oral suspension. The suspension contains a preservative to minimise the possibility of harmful microbial growth. To assure uniform mixing, gently invert the NVP suspension bottle several times. Do not shake the bottle vigorously.

Administer NVP suspension orally using a calibrated oral syringe or a hypodermic syringe after removing the needle. The syringe should hold a maximum volume of 3 ml or less to ensure accuracy. Since multiple patients will receive medication from the same bottle of NVP suspension, measure the suspension by pouring up to 1 ml into a clean medicine cup. Then draw it into the syringe without using a needle and administer it orally. Do not return the remainder of the NVP in the cup to the bottle; discard it.

Ideally, use a new syringe for each patient. Discard used syringes to avoid contamination of the NVP multiple dose bottle and the spread of infections between patients. If a new syringe is not available, clean and disinfect the used syringe as follows:

i) Wash in clean soapy water (draw soapy water up into the syringe, using the plunger),
ii) Rinse thoroughly with filtered water (draw filtered water several times into the syringe, until clear),
iii) Allow to air dry, with plunger removed, on a clean surface.

Never give NVP with any syringes that have previously been used to give injections.

CARE DURING ANTENATAL, LABOUR, DELIVERY, AND POSTPARTUM PERIODS

One of the specific interventions for PMTCT is the adoption of safer obstetric practices, within the context of basic prenatal, peripartum, and postnatal care.

Antenatal Care

All mothers, and particularly HIV-infected mothers, get basic antenatal care (ANC). In addition to regular follow-up for pregnancy monitoring, this includes the following:

i) *Malaria Intermittent Preventive Therapy (IPT):* Recent studies have shown that malaria may increase the risk of HIV transmission from mother to baby. WHO recommends intermittent treatment for prevention of adverse effects of malaria infection during pregnancy for women in highly endemic areas. In areas of chloroquine resistance, sulfadoxine-pyrimethamine 500/25mg (SP or Fansidar) is now recommended as the alternative anti-malarial drugs. For such areas, WHO recommends Fansidar for malaria prophylaxis in pregnancy. The dose is 3 tabs of Fansidar as early as possible in the second trimester (from 13-28 weeks) and 3 tabs early in the third trimester (from 29-36 weeks). Do not give Fansidar (or any other sulfa drug) within four weeks of estimated date of delivery (EDD), because it may cause neonatal jaundice. This regimen is cheaper and more efficacious than chloroquine.

ii) *Nutrition and pregnancy*
- Provide nutrition counselling
- Give iron/folate, one capsule/tablet two times per day for the treatment of anaemia.
- Give iron/folate routinely for all pregnant, postpartum, and post-abortion women, one capsule/tablet one time per day, in pregnancy.

— Continue up to 3 months after delivery or abortion.

Give Vitamin A 200,000 IU capsule two times within six weeks of delivery.

— De-worm with mebendazole 5 tablets, single dose in second trimester.

— Give multivitamin supplementation if feasible.

iii) *STI Screening and Treatment:* Treat STIs according to national guidelines. Syphilis screening and treatment for the woman and her partner are offered as part of routine ANC in most facilities.

iv) *Tetanus Immunisation*

Vaccinate all women (HIV-positive, -negative, or unknown status) with tetanus toxoid vaccine following the national guidelines.

v) *TB, HIV, and Pregnancy:* During antenatal clinic or admission in labour, the antenatal clinic nurse, the HIV counsellor, or the OB ward nurse or midwife should question all HIV-positive mothers for TB symptoms. For all antenatal or peripartum patients with symptoms suggestive of active pulmonary TB (cough for >3 weeks, blood in sputum, night sweats, fever, weight loss, etc.):

— Use respiratory isolation precautions.

— Collect 3 sputa for AFB.

— Consult physician and/or TB control officer/coordinator.

— If the sputa are negative, obtain a chest X-ray (with appropriate shielding to protect the fetus).

— Apply a TB skin test, if tuberculin is available.

During antenatal clinic or admission in labour, apply TB skin tests (0.1 cc of tuberculin intradermally on the forearm) on all HIV-positive mothers who have not previously been tested, if tuberculin is available. For those who have a positive test (5 mm or greater in duration at 48-72 hours), evaluate for latent or active TB with a chest X-ray. Healthy women with a negative skin test result (less than 5 mm) do not need therapy or chest X-ray.

Sick women with symptoms of advanced AIDS may have a false negative TB skin test. For these women, consult physician and/or TB control officer/coordinator, if you suspect active TB. For patients with abnormal chest X-rays suggestive of active TB, collect 3 sputa for AFB and consult physician for medical evaluation. Consider signs and symptoms of extrapulmonary TB, such as adenopathy (possibly TB adenitis), meningitis, etc., if HIV-positive patients become ill. Extrapulmonary forms of TB are more common in HIV-positive persons.

For latent TB infection (positive TB skin test with no symptoms of active disease and no chest X-ray findings suggestive of active TB):

— WHO recommends prophylaxis (protection against later development of active disease) with nine months of isoniasid (INH). The dose is 300 mg daily or 900 mg directly observed treatment (DOT) two times per week and pyridoxine (25 mg) daily or two times per week with monthly follow-up to monitor for toxicity.

— Before starting INH prophylaxis, assess whether the patient is willing and able to complete the full nine-month course. It is better not to start than to stop before completing the full course, because partial treatment may lead to drug resistance.

— If the patient is likely to adhere to the full course, begin INH at the time of the postpartum hospital discharge or in the third trimester of pregnancy.

vi) *Maternal Health Assessment:* Thoroughly examine all HIV-positive pregnant or postpartum women, obtain a baseline hemoglobin, white blood cell count and differential, and erythrocyte sedimentation rate (ESR). Record the results on the follow-up register. Calculate the total lymphocyte count (TLC) by multiplying the WBC by the proportion of lymphocytes in the differential count.

vii) *Prophylaxis for Pneumocystis carinii Pneumonia (PCP)*: Offer mothers who meet the following clinical and/or laboratory criteria PCP prophylaxis with trimethoprim-sulfamethoxazole (TMP/SMX), also known as Bactrim or Cotrimoxazole:

— Asymptomatic with a Total Lymphocyte Count (TLC) <2,000/μL

— WHO Clinical Stage II, III, or IV disease.

The appropriate prophylactic dose of TMP/SMX is two single strength (TMP 80 mg/SMX 400 mg) tabs daily. Do not give TMP/SMX to women at >36 weeks gestation due to its potential for causing jaundice, and possibly kernicterus, in the newborn. In addition, TMP/SMX prophylaxis is recommended for HIV-exposed infants at >6 weeks of age.

Labour and Delivery

i) *Cesarean Section Option:* Delivery by Caesarian section (C/S) reduces the transmission of HIV from mother to child by about 50 per cent. In many countries, HIV-positive mothers routinely deliver by C/S, but in most facilities in resource-poor settings, C/Ss are not available, are prohibitively expensive, and have high risks of morbidity and mortality. For these reasons, C/Ss are not done routinely for deliveries of HIV-positive mothers in such settings. In facilities that can perform C/Ss with minimal morbidity and mortality, offer C/S to HIV-positive antenatal patients who can afford to pay for it. For such patients, schedule elective C/Ss for women after 38 weeks, if estimated date of delivery (EDD) is well documented.

ii) *Universal precautions:* Midwives and maternity staff should practice universal precautions when handling blood and body fluids from all women during labour and delivery.

iii) *Counselling/NVP administration:*

a) For mothers identified as HIV-positive, verify labour and ask the mother whether she took her NVP. If NVP was not taken, provide another tablet.

b) Some mothers may know their status from previous testing. Offer NVP if they say they are HIV-positive.

c) Offer VTC to women in labour whose HIV status is unknown. Offer NVP if the first rapid test is positive. The second rapid test and further counselling can be done after delivery. Since NVP has proven efficacy, is a WHO standard treatment, and no longer requires written informed consent to administer, the risk to the baby of not giving it outweighs the concern that the labouring woman is unable to give informed consent.

iv) *Vaginal delivery-avoid*

a) Artificial rupture of membranes before late second stage.

b) Continuing labor for more than three hours after rupture of membranes (ROM) if C/S is available quickly. Allowing labor to continue after ROM results in greater exposure of the baby to maternal blood and vaginal secretions and greater risk of HIV transmission. If C/S is not available quickly, avoid unnecessary vaginal examinations after ROM.

c) Unnecessary episiotomy, which will increase the baby's exposure to maternal blood.

d) Unnecessary instrumentation (e.g., forceps, vacuum extraction, scalp electrodes, electrical suctioning of infant's nares) that will potentially cause open wounds on the mother or baby or otherwise increase the transfer of maternal blood to the baby. However, this should not prevent delivery staff from performing such instrumentation if necessary: e.g., use forceps or vacuum for true fetal distress and electrical suction or intubation for meconium aspiration.

e) Multiple vaginal examinations, and examinations by multiple providers.

f) Prolonged obstructed labour, by monitoring labor carefully and intervening appropriately when labour is prolonged (i.e., augmentation of labour or C/S). Plot the course of labor on a labour progress/time curve to determine if labour is progressing normally. These practices are good obstetric care for all women, but are particularly important for HIV-positive women.

Immediate Postnatal Care

When the infant is born:

i) Dry the blood and maternal secretions off the baby.
ii) Avoid unnecessary or aggressive nasal suction.
iii) Weigh the baby and record the birth weight on the growth chart on the "Road to Health" card. The mother brings this card to each well infant visit to record immunisations and development.
iv) If the mother has chosen to breast-feed, put the infant to the breast within 30 minutes. Ensure proper positioning and latching on. This is especially important for new mothers who have no prior experience with breast-feeding.
v) If the mother has chosen not to breast-feed, ensure that she has brought with her all needed supplies for replacement feeding.

Continuing Neonatal Care

Administer NVP syrup before discharge. Provide the infants' first immunisations and record on the "Road to Health" card. Comply with national immunisation guidelines. Ensure that the mother is well. If she is sick, refer her for medical evaluation. Before discharge, schedule follow-up visit for mother and infant to see you.

COUNSELLING FOR SAFER INFANT FEEDING

When an HIV-positive woman breast-feeds her infant, a further 5-20 per cent risk of transmission is added. Among 672 infants (HIV-negative at birth) born to HIV-positive mothers in Malawi, 47 (7 per cent) seroconverted while breast-feeding. The cumulative infection rate while breast-feeding at 5, 11, 17, and 23 months was 3.5 per cent, 7.0 per cent, 8.9 per cent, and 10.3 per cent, respectively. Monthly incidence was 0.7 per cent from 1-5 months, 0.6 per cent from 6-11 months, and 0.3 per cent from 12-17 months.

Thus, the risk for breast milk transmission is the highest in the early months of life the time when infants are most susceptible to morbidity from enteric infections from contaminated feeds. This has created a public health dilemma in resource-constrained settings, where breast-feeding is the primary guarantee for child health, development, and survival, particularly in the early months of life.

Replacement feeding means the process of feeding a child who is not receiving any breast milk with a diet that provides all the nutrients the child needs. During the first six months this should be with a suitable BMS-commercial formula, or home-prepared formula with micronutrient supplements.

After six months, preferably feed a suitable BMS, and complementary foods made from appropriately prepared and nutrient-enriched family foods, given four times a day. If suitable BMSs are not available, feed appropriately prepared family foods that are further enriched, given four times a day. Breast-feeding and feeding BMSs at the same time (mixed feeding) is the most dangerous option for the baby. This practice exposes the baby to all the disadvantages of replacement feeding as well as increased risk of HIV infection from breast milk.

Breast-feeding

In most developing countries breast-feeding is nearly universal and is the normative infant feeding method.

The major benefits of breast-feeding are given below.

i) reduces infant morbidity and mortality associated with infectious diseases, particularly diarrhoea and respiratory infections. This is especially important for younger infants of women who are more disadvantaged and have less education. These infants may experience up to five to six times more illness and death from diarrhoea, respiratory infections, and other infectious disease in the absence of breast-feeding.

ii) provides perfect nutrition and is the natural food for newborns and young infants.

iii) bonds mother and child.

iv) inexpensive and readily available.

v) stimulates uterine contractions immediately postpartum, thus helping to stop postpartum bleeding and stimulates uterine involution (shrinking to pre-pregnant size) in the first few weeks postpartum.

vi) benefits the mother by birth spacing, facilitating involution of the uterus after delivery, hence reducing the risk of postpartum haemorrhage, and protecting against certain cancers.

Some disadvantages of breast-feeding are:

i) Risk of postnatal transmission of HIV.

ii) Only the mother can feed the baby (unless a suitable wet nurse is available).

iii) May increase maternal mortality rate in HIV-infected mothers.

Factors that increase HIV transmission from mother-to-child are:

i) Seroconversion (acquiring initial infection) during lactation

ii) Bleeding or cracked nipples
iii) Subclinical and clinical mastitis
iv) Breast abscesses
v) Mixed feeding
vi) Open sores in infant's mouth

This highlights the need for proper instruction of mothers in good breast-feeding techniques, the practice of exclusive breast-feeding, prompt treatment for breast conditions, and avoidance of HIV infection for those who are not infected, or whose status is unknown. This enables HIV-infected mothers who choose to breast-feed, and those whose status is unknown, to breast-feed optimally with less risk of HIV transmission through breast milk.

Some guidance on optimal breast-feeding for mothers are given below:

i) *If the baby is not positioned correctly*
   — Baby's tummy is not flat against mother's
   Show the mother correct positioning
   — Baby is facing mother and is close to her.
   — Baby's tummy is flat against mother's tummy.
ii) *If not properly attached to the breast*
   — Baby looks like it is sucking a straw.
   — Baby's mouth does not cover areola.
   Show the mother correct attachment
   — Baby's chin is touching the breast.
   — Baby's mouth covers all the areola (dark skin around the nipple).
   — Baby's lower lip is curled outward.

An HIV-positive mother who chooses to breast-feed should be supported to maintain exclusive breast-feeding and to wean her infant early (no later than six months). As much as possible, a period of mixed feeding should be avoided or kept to the absolute minimum through "rapid weaning."

Weaning and Reducing Breast Engorgement

"Abrupt weaning" can cause the baby to be fussy and to feed poorly, and cause the mother to have painful breast engorgement. Breast engorgement can lead to plugged milk ducts, mastitis, and breast abscesses, if not treated correctly. One must balance the danger of increased HIV transmission from brief mixed feeding against the risks of poor feeding and breast engorgement from abrupt weaning. Therefore, it may be most acceptable to wean over the course of about two weeks (rapid weaning). Although abrupt weaning is optimal practice, it is advisable to work with each mother to achieve weaning safely over as short a time as possible.

Rapid Weaning

i) Express breast milk and give to baby using a cup, especially during the day.

ii) At first, continue to breast-feed during the night, to assure adequate rest for mother and baby.

iii) Increase the number of expressed breast milk feeds from the cup, while decreasing the number of feeds directly from the breast gradually over a two-week period.

iv) Learn how to prepare animal milk or commercial infant formula

v) Stop breast-feeding as soon as possible when the baby is used to feeding from the cup.

vi) Introduce complementary foods when baby is six months old.

Reducing Breast Engorgement in Abrupt or Rapid Weaning

i) *Do*: Wear a bra or breast binder that presses firmly against the nipples. It may help to put gauze or clean cloth over the nipples, under the bra cup or breast binder, to absorb dripping milk and add pressure on the nipples. If engorgement is severe or painful, briefly remove or loosen bra or binder and allow milk to drip, unstimulated. In extreme cases, it may be necessary to express a small amount of milk. Use mild analgesics, such as paracetamol, aspirin, or ibuprofen as needed for pain.

ii) Taking combination estrogen/progesterone birth control pills may decrease milk production in mothers who are trying to wean. However, starting combination birth control pills prior to two-three weeks postpartum is not recommended, because the estrogen may slightly increase the mother's hypercoagulable state.

iii) Some have suggested applying washed cabbage leaves over the breasts, under the bra or binder, changing them twice a day, and leaving the nipple free. There is insufficient evidence for or against the effectiveness of this method.

iv) *Do not*: Use any type of nipple stimulation (squeezing, sucking, massaging), as this will promote lactation.

v) *Do not*: Reduce fluid intake or take diuretics, as this is dangerous to the mother, especially in the immediate postpartum period or if she has been working or engaging in vigorous physical activity.

Women Choosing Not to Breast-feed-Replacement Feeding

i) Due to the complexity of the issues involved, counsel all HIV-infected mothers about the risks and benefits of various infant feeding options and provide specific guidance in selecting the most suitable option.

ii) When replacement feeding is acceptable, feasible, affordable, sustainable, and safe, WHO recommends that all HIV infected mothers not breast-feed. Otherwise, exclusive breast-feeding is recommended during the first six months of life.

iii) To minimize the risk of HIV transmission, breast-feeding should be discontinued as soon as feasible, taking into account local circumstances, the individual woman's situation, and the risks of replacement feeding (including infections other than HIV and malnutrition)

Table 3

Guidance on breast milk substitutes and modified breast-feeding

Breast milk substitutes	
Options	*Requirements*
Commercial baby formula	Financial means for 20 kg of powdered milk or 44 tins of 450g or 40 tins of 500 g: (80,000 CFAs or US$133) for 6 months. Potable water and adequate level of education.
Animal milk	Whole animal milk not recommended before age 12 months. Modified animal milk not ideal, but sometimes is the only option
Modified Breast-feeding	
Early discontinuation of breast-feeding (especially important in mothers with AIDS or TB)	Optimal date of cessation determined. Every mother wanting to stop must have substitute available.
Heating of breast milk to 62.5°C for 30 minutes	Pasteurized milk of higher nutritive value than others. Disadvantage: Destroys immune globulins that would protect the baby against infection. Highly motivated mother required.
Feeding by a wet nurse	HIV-negative wet nurse fully informed of baby's HIV status and of possible risk of infection in case of nipple cracks, if baby is HIV-positive.

Caveats on Replacement Feeding

i) Powdered, commercially made infant formula
   a) Lacks protective maternal immunoglobulins.

ii) Heat-treated (pasteurised) expressed breast milk from the mother
   a) May lose some immunoglobulins during pasteurisation process.
   b) Experience from South Africa and Zimbabwe shows that heating breast milk is technically very demanding and difficult, and would take an exceptional mother to adhere to this modification of breast-feeding.

iii) Breast milk from an uninfected wet nurse.
   a) Wet nurses who are willing to be tested for HIV may be difficult to find.

iv) Animal milk
   a) Whole, unmodified cow milk is not recommended before age 12 months, because of its high solute load, low iron content, and risk of causing intestinal bleeding, leading to anaemia.
   b) Modified animal milk, diluted with water and with added sugar, lacks iron, zinc, and other essential micronutrients. More research is needed to determine the effect on growth and nutritional adequacy, especially before age six months.
   c) Consider animal milk pre-diluted by a vendor to be unsafe, unless the mother is sure the vendor follows the instructions below.

Counselling Mothers on Replacement Feeding

i) *Time*: Begin counselling HIV-positive mothers on infant feeding options either at the time you inform them of a positive test result or soon thereafter, and continue counselling on each subsequent antenatal visit. If a mother who plans not to breast-feed has just delivered, counsel her and, if possible, other family members before she leaves the hospital. If she is already breast-feeding, determine when she plans to stop. Ask if this is a good time to discuss replacement feeding.

ii) *Place*: (ideally, counselling should occur in a setting where you can demonstrate food preparation techniques):

   a) In private counselling room in clinic

   b) During home visit

   c) During support group meetings

iii) Feasibility:

   a) Will she leave her baby in care of someone else while she goes to work?

   b) Is there a responsible baby carer who will be able to safely prepare replacement feeds?

   c) Can she afford replacement feeds?

   d) Are adequate firewood, water sources, and dishes available to prepare boiled water and clean containers?

iv). Type of replacement feed available in her local community:

   a) Commercial infant formula.

   b) Animal milk (use whole milk, not milk diluted by vendor).

   c) Liquid porridge. Most such preparations are nutritionally inadequate as a sole food source.

v) *Traditional practices*: It is critical to make counselling as culturally appropriate as possible, to take advantage of helpful practices, and to find culturally sensitive ways of discouraging harmful practices:

   a) Is mixed feeding the norm, especially when the mother returns to work on their farms?

   b) Is liquid porridge commonly given to infants? Animal milk?

c) Are foods softened by premastication or other techniques to add nutrients to infant feeds? Are infants given liquid from boiled foods, such as stews?

d) Is wet-nursing practised? Are there certain women designated to be wet nurses?

e) If there a customary carer (e.g., mother-in-law), and has the mother disclosed her HIV status?

Preparing Animal Milk

Although animal milk is not ideal, it is the only option for many mothers. When possible, additional sources of vitamins and minerals should be added.

i) Have ready the following materials:

a) Fresh, clean animal milk

b) Boiled, clean water (potable water)

c) 2-liter jar with a tight cover

d) 2 cups without covers

e) 1 larger, clear, marked container to measure 100 mls

f) 1 teaspoon

g) Clean mat or other material on which to place the clean utensils

h) 2 teaspoonfuls of sugar for each feeding

ii). Have the mother prepare the milk as below. Explain, observe, correct errors, praise success.

a) If she uses undiluted, fresh cow, goat, or camel milk:

— Wash hands and utensils with soap and clean water.

— Measure 100 ml of milk.

— Put the milk into a clean jug.

— Add 50 ml of clean, boiled water that has cooled.

— Add 2 teaspoonfuls of sugar.

— Mix and boil the milk.

— Let the milk cool.

— Measure the amount to feed the baby.

b) If she uses undiluted, fresh sheep or buffalo milk, modify the process:

— Measure 50 ml of milk.

— Add 50 ml of potable cool water.

— Add 1 teaspoon of sugar.

Preparing Commercial Infant Formula

i) Follow instructions on formula package.

ii) Prepare clean boiled water and utensils

Advantages of Replacement Feeding

i) May reduce maternal mortality.

ii) Eliminates the risk of HIV infection to the baby through breast milk.

iii) The infant can be fed by someone else.

Disadvantages of Replacement Feeding

i) Carries other health risks for the baby, especially if feeding involves the use of feeding bottles and unsafe water or if formula is mixed incorrectly due to inability to comprehend instructions.

ii) May lead to rationing because of the cost of formula, fuel, soap, thermos, cup, spoon, and other supplies.

iii) Illness and death from diarrhoea, respiratory problems, and other infectious diseases is up to five or six times higher in the first two months of an infant's life when not breast-fed

iv) Discrimination toward the mother by family and community, and possible inadvertent disclosure of HIV status.

Making Replacement Feeding Easier and Safer

i) For each mother giving breast milk substitutes, explain how to use a cup to feed her baby. Mention that using a spoon to feed the baby is too slow and may discourage the mother and baby.

ii) Tell the mother to feed the baby using an open cup following the steps below:

Step 1: Hold the baby upright or almost upright on your lap.

Step 2: Hold the cup of milk to the baby's lips.

Step 3: Rest the cup lightly on the baby's bottom lip.

Step 4: Tilt the cup so that the milk just reaches the baby's lips.

Step 5: Hold the cup to the baby's lips and let the baby take the milk at his or her own pace.

Do not pour the milk into the baby's mouth

iii) Observe the mother and correct any errors.

iv) Talk to the mother about how to prepare the breast milk substitute of choice. The health worker should refer to the instructions for preparation provided for commercial formulae. If the mother feeds the infant animal milk, use pasteurized or heat-treated milk.

Infant Feeding Guidelines

A variety of tools have been developed to help a counsellor guide a mother in making an infant feeding choice. The following table summarizes common health worker guidelines for mothers with different HIV statuses.

Table 4

HIV and Infant feeding counselling guidelines in resource-poor communities

Situation	*Health worker guidelines*
Mother's status is unknown	Promote availability and use of confidential testing. Promote breast-feeding as safer than artificial feeding. Teach mother how to avoid exposure to HIV.
HIV-negative mother	Promote breast-feeding as safest infant feeding method (exclusive breast-feeding for first 6 months. introduction of appropriate complementary foods at about 6 months. and continued breast-feeding up to 24 months and beyond). Teach mother how to avoid exposure to HIV.
HIV-positive mother who is considering her feeding options	Treat with ARV drugs if feasible. Counsel mother on the safety, availability, and affordability of feasible infant feeding options. Help mother choose and provide safest available infant feeding methods. Teach mother how to avoid sexual transmission of HIV.
HIV-positive mother who chooses to breast-feed	Promote safer breast-feeding (exclusive breast-feeding for 3 to 6 months, prevention and treatment of breast problems of mothers and thrush in infants, and shortened duration of breast-feeding when replacements are safe and feasible). Treat with ARV drugs if feasible.
HIV-positive mother who chooses to feed artificially	Help mother choose the safest alternative infant feeding strategy (methods, timing, etc.). Support her in her choice (provide education on hygienic preparation, health care, family planning services, etc.).

Often, a mother's infant feeding choice will change over time, as she resolves conflicts between what she would like to do and what her circumstances dictate. A counsellor's role is to provide information on all options, guide the mother in making her choice, and support her in her choice.

The infant feeding counselling should be done in PMTCT programmes:

— During group health discussions. It should include addressing maternal nutrition issues and breast care to prepare mothers for exclusive breast-feeding.

— During post-test counselling positive women and refer to the Cato Manor tool for facilitating infant feeding choice. During early labour as appropriate for HIV-positive women. In particular it is important to affirm the mother's feeding method of choice, and specifically to make sure she has everything needed for replacement feeding, if she does not intend to breast-feed.

— After delivery to support the mother in initiating her feeding choice. Mothers who choose to breast-feed should put their infants to the breast within 30 minutes of delivery.

— At follow-up clinic visits and during home visits to sustain/ adhere to the feeding method of choice.

— Ongoing to avoid mixed feeding, by supporting the process of rapid weaning for breast-feeding mothers, and to promote the safe introduction of other appropriate foods for all mothers. Encourage HIV-positive mothers whose infants test HIV-negative (6 weeks PCR) to wean their infants as soon as possible after three months, and no later than six months.

— Provide mothers with subsequent opportunities beyond the initial counselling to ask questions and to revisit their choice. Support them to follow through with their choices.

CARING FOR AN INFANT OF AN HIV-POSITIVE MOTHER

Infants of HIV-positive mothers require regular follow-up and care. Their mothers and families need information on how to take care of their infants, and particularly how to make full use of the regular infant welfare clinics for growth monitoring and immunisations. The following information will help you guide the mothers when they have questions.

Maternal antibodies of the IgG type cross the placenta. Therefore, HIV antibodies will be detected among all infants born to HIV-positive mothers in the first months of life and up to 15 months of age. An HIV antibody test is therefore not a good way to determine which infant has been truly infected and which one is just reflecting maternal antibodies.

For this reason, infant HIV diagnosis requires a special test called the Polymerase Chain Reaction (PCR), which detects the virus (or components of it) rather than the antibodies. However, the test is very expensive, difficult to perform, and available only in sophisticated labs and research centers.

However, for breast-fed babies, the definitive test is one performed at least three months after the baby is weaned, and preferably six months after weaning. This schedule outlines the timing of these tests and emphasizes the importance of pre-and post-test counselling for infant testing. In the absence of HIV PCR tests, obtain an HIV antibody test such as an HIV rapid test (or ELISA) when the infant is 15-18 months of age, at least three months after weaning. As much as possible, coordinate follow-up visits within the existing immunisation schedule, unless infants need to return for "sick" visits.

PMTCT Follow-Up Protocol for Infants of HIV-Positive Mothers

Newborn

— Give BCG Vaccine and Oral Polio Vaccine (OPV) prior to discharge for all babies. If these immunisations are not given shortly after birth, give them at the earliest opportunity thereafter or at the 6-week visit. On "Road to Health" card, record "NVP given" date(s). "Collect blood for PCR at 6 weeks," and Birth weight. Stamp the infant's card with the SPC (special prenatal care) stamp, and give mother an appointment slip.

6 weeks:

— Measure and chart the infant's weight and length on the "Road to Health" card.

— Immunize. If BCG was not given at birth, give it now. Collect blot specimen for PCR.

— Do not write the patient's name on the blot paper.

— Write out date of collection and date of birth.

— UNAIDS recommends trimethoprim/sulfamethoxazole (TMP/SMX) (trade names: Cotrimoxazole, Bactrim, or Septra) prophylaxis from six weeks through 15 months of age for all HIV-exposed infants. If cost is an issue, give priority to all PCR-positive and all symptomatic infants. For HIV-positive infants, continue PCP prophylaxis if child has clinical signs of immunosuppression or if CD4 count is <500 or CD4 per cent is <15 per cent. It protects against Pneumocystis carinii pneumonia (PCP), a common opportunistic infection that causes severe pneumonia, especially among young infants, and has been found to be fairly common in Cote d'Ivoire, Malawi, and Uganda. TMP/SMX prophylaxis also protects against common bacterial infections including ear and urinary tract infections. Further studies are needed to determine the cost effectiveness of PCP prophylaxis in HIV-exposed infants, and some investigators recommend stopping treatment at six months of age.

— Concerns have been raised that, although UNAIDS recommends PCP prophylaxis for all infants of HIV-positive mothers, only about 15 per cent of NVP-treated babies will be infected with HIV. Thus, about 85 per cent of babies receive prophylaxis needlessly. Also, treating so many babies with prophylactic antibiotics may lead to resistance to TMP/SMX, making it less useful for treating sick patients. Thus, each PMTCT site will need to decide whether or not to provide PCP prophylaxis for babies of HIV-positive mothers.

— If PCR testing is available at six weeks of age, give prophylaxis only to those babies who are PCR-positive. If your programme offers PCP prophylaxis, provide it to all HIV-exposed infants with whom you have regular contact and closely monitor adherence in those infants whose mothers agree to give them prophylaxis.

Six months to 12 months

— Measure and chart the infant's weight and length on the growth chart in "Road to Health" card.

— Give measles vaccine-first dose. Repeat measles vaccine at the age of nine months.

— Make sure that any missed DPT and OPV vaccines are given to ensure that each infant receives all doses of each vaccine.

— Women who decide to breast-feed their babies should wean the infant rapidly at 6 months, if not sooner. Facilitate this process of rapid weaning.

15 months +

— Measure and chart the infant's weight and length growth chart on the "Road to Health" card.

— Perform a rapid HIV antibody test to determine the infant's HIV status. If the baby stopped breast-feeding three months, or preferably six months, prior to the antibody test, or has never breast-fed, this is the infant's definitive diagnostic test.

— If an infant who is still breast-feeding at this age tests HIV-negative, actively encourage and support the mother to stop breast-feeding.

Immunisations for Infants of HIV-Positive Mothers

The following table displays the recommended schedule of vaccinations for infants of HIV-positive mothers.

Table 5

Recommended Use of Vaccines and Immune Globulins in Persons with Altered Immunocompetence

Vaccine	*Asymptomatic HIV Infection*	*Symptomatic HIV Infection*	*Optimal Timing of Immunisation*
BCG*	Yes	No	Birth
DPT	Yes	Yes	6,10,14 weeks
OPV**	Yes	Yes	0, 6, 10, 14 weeks
Measles	Yes	Yes	6 and 9 months
Hepatitis B	Yes	Yes	As for uninfected children
Yellow fever	Yes	No	
Tetanus toxoid	Yes	Yes	

*Newborns (including those born to HIV-positive women MUST receive BCG at birth. At this time, infants born to HIV-positive women are without symptoms).

**Infants and under fives who were perinatally exposed to HIV should receive OPV during national vaccination drives.

Infant Welfare/Well-Child Care

— Weigh, measure length, and monitor growth to detect "failure to thrive" and malnutrition. Record and chart weights and lengths at each visit on the "Road To Health" card. Interpret the growth trend to the mother and intervene as needed. Give mothers ongoing infant feeding, weaning, and nutrition education and counselling. It is better to prevent than to treat HIV-related malnutrition because severe forms are difficult to reverse.

— Discuss basic hygiene issues, including hand washing, proper food preparation, proper cleaning of spilled body fluids, personal cleanliness, etc.

— Provide vitamin A supplementation according to national schedule.
— De-worm children every three-six months, especially when the child begins to walk and to eat raw fruits and vegetables.
— Treat any incidental illnesses promptly.

CARING OF HIV-POSITIVE MOTHER

When a person learns he/she is HIV positive, it is a life changing experience. It is particularly difficult for a pregnant woman who is well to discover that she is HIV positive. In addition to worrying about her own health, the expecting mother is burdened with the possibility of passing the infection to her infant. Encourage and support every woman with HIV to "live positively" with her condition. Positive living is about having a positive attitude, confidence that you can manage your circumstances, and the knowledge and skills to do so. Positive living helps not only the woman, but also her family and friends.

Follow-up of HIV-positive women and their infants is critical to provide ongoing primary care and support, as well as HIV-related care, should they become symptomatic. As much as possible, coordinate these follow-up visits with the infants' immunisation schedules, unless they need specific HIV-related care or are not well. A six week visit is normally scheduled for mothers who have uncomplicated vaginal deliveries.

Most women diagnosed through the PMTCT programmes are quite healthy and have no, or few, symptoms. There are things that each mother can do to maintain or improve her health. These include:

— Eating a balanced diet. Cooking meats and eggs thoroughly and washing fruits and raw vegetables with potable water or treated water.

— Maintaining good personal hygiene including particular attention to oral hygiene, fingernails and toenails, and private areas.

— Getting immediate and proper treatment for every infection or illness.

— Avoiding drinking alcohol and smoking cigarettes.

— Using birth control to avoid unintended pregnancies or delay future pregnancies.

— *Practising safer sex*. Using condoms consistently and regularly to avoid reinfection or infecting a partner, and avoiding sex during menses or when either partner has symptoms of a sexually transmitted infection (STI). Getting STIs treated promptly. Preventing malaria infection through the use of impregnated bed nets, clearing bushes around the house, getting rid of stagnant water, etc.

— Balancing exercise and rest (most women's regular daily work schedule is exercise enough, but they need to rest and at least 8 hours' sleep at night). Accepting her condition and understanding the implications.

— Obtaining medical care promptly when she gets sick.

— Working toward disclosing her status to her partner and family.

— Planning for the future of her children and family (succession planning) including will-making.

— Taking care of herself mentally and spiritually by obtaining regular counselling, participating in a support group (if available), and seeking support from her church and family.

— Continuing to participate in community activities.

— Developing or consolidating her support network and participating in a support group for HIV-positive women.

— Challenging stigma and discrimination against persons living with HIV/AIDS.

Family Planning Counselling and Services

Offer every PMTCT client and her partner family planning (FP) counselling and services. For antenatal clients, start at the first ANC visit and follow up with additional information at subsequent visits. Explain the importance of child-spacing, in order to preserve the health of the mother and the financial security of the family. Provide verbal and, when applicable, written information and education on all FP options available at your facility and your referral facilities. If your facility does not already have FP protocols and patient education information, work with other health providers to develop these materials.

It is important for PMTCT programmes to closely coordinate with FP programmes, as well as with maternal and child health and obstetric programmes, in order to provide optimal care. If it is possible for your facility to acquire condoms at no charge, offer them to all clients at no charge and in adequate supply. Give highest priority to providing condoms at no charge to all HIV support group members. If other FP methods are available, offer them at the lowest cost possible to the clients, within the capability of your facility's fiscal status. If more effective FP methods are not available, the facility must at least offer thorough education on use of the rhythm method and on avoidance of "country medicine" or hearsay "methods" that do not work.

For HIV-infected individuals, explain that subsequent pregnancies may further stress their immune system and possibly advance their progression toward AIDS. Explain that, with each subsequent pregnancy, they will again risk passing on HIV to their babies. Although condoms, when used consistently and correctly, offer dual protection against HIV and pregnancy, they are not 100 per cent effective against either. Therefore, encourage all such patients to use "safer sex" and the "A" and "B" of the "ABCs," in addition to using condoms, to prevent HIV transmission. Also, encourage them to use a second family planning method, when possible, to prevent subsequent pregnancies. The PMTCT Programme will, as resources permit, attempt to subsidize FP methods, including sterilisation, for all HIV-positive clients.

Seek to use longer term, sustainable contraceptive methods for women (especially HIV-positive women) who desire no further pregnancies, but for whom sterilisation is not an option. For example, Depo-provera or intrauterine devices (IUDs) may be more cost-effective than oral contraceptive pills (OCPs) because of their longer duration of action and reduced need for daily motivation.

IUDs are contraindicated for women who do not follow the ABCs of HIV prevention and are therefore at risk of acquiring sexually transmitted infections (STIs), because IUDs may enable STIs to ascend to the upper genital tract, where such infections can cause pelvic inflammatory disease (PID). IUDs are relatively (not absolutely) contraindicated in all HIV-positive women, who are at increased risk of PID from opportunistic infections.

The counsellor must give enough information on the mechanism of action, efficacy, and cost of available methods for the client to weigh the risks and benefits of the various methods in relation to her/his own health needs and financial status. Once the client decides to use FP, it is the counsellor's responsibility to either explain the methods in adequate detail to enable correct use or refer the client to an experienced FP provider who can further explain and provide the requested method.

Support Groups

Mothers who have not joined support groups should have the opportunity to do so at any time during follow-up. Support groups provide opportunities for ongoing support, information/education, skills building, peer support and encouragement, and follow-up medical care for HIV-positive mothers and their babies. Consider forming support groups for the fathers as well.

Nutrition

Eating a balanced diet is very important for HIV-positive mothers and especially for those who are breast-feeding. Breast-feeding mothers should continue prenatal vitamins, including folate and iron, and if possible should have an extra meal a day.

Nutrition counselling is especially important for persons living with HIV/AIDS, caregivers, family members, and HIV-exposed or -infected infants and children. HIV/AIDS and malnutrition are closely interrelated. HIV infection causes malnutrition through multiple mechanisms:

— Negative impact on food intake
— Losses through diarrhoea and vomiting
— Reduction of nutrient absorption
— Increase of energy requirements

There is some evidence that malnutrition, particularly vitamin A deficiency, may increase MTCT rates. Recommendations for nutrition counselling and care for people with HIV/AIDS vary with the nutritional status and stage of the disease. Recommendations at the asymptomatic stage focus on counselling about good nutrition and a healthy diet. The recommendation should take into account locally available foods and the need for increased energy intakes.

With disease progression, dietary modification may be required to maintain food intake and absorption at volumes as near normal as possible. In addition, if the health of a lactating mother is failing, actively encourage and support the mother to stop breast-feeding. Not only might this be beneficial for the mother's health as suggested by one study, but, with failing health and a higher viral load, the risk of postnatal transmission through breast milk becomes higher.

Opportunistic Infections

Opportunistic infections (OIs) are those diseases that do not cause sickness in persons with normal immunity but do so in people whose immunity is compromised. For each OI, there are specific drugs that are used to cure, treat, or alleviate symptoms. Refer the client to a doctor for proper medical treatment, if an OI is suspected. The table below shows selected common OIs.

Table 6. Common HIV-related opportunistic infections

Name	*Description*
Pneumocystis carinii pneumonia	– A protozoal infection that can cause a fatal pneumonia. – Early symptoms include fatigue and shortness of breath. As the infection intensifies, rapid breathing, dry cough, fever, chills, night sweats, and weight loss occur. – Consider prophylaxis with TMP/SMZ. Treatment is with IV or oral TMP/SMZ.
Cryptococcus meningitis	– This fungal infection causes an inflammation of the covering of the spinal cord and brain. – Symptoms include fever, blurred vision with photophobia (eyes sensitive to light), mental confusion, very severe headache, and a stiff or aching neck. Tuberculosis A bacterial infection that attacks the lungs and other organs and can cause meningitis. – Consider TB in everyone with HIV. Symptoms include fatigue, fever, night sweats, weight loss, and a prolonged cough producing sputum and sometimes blood. – Consider screening with tuberculin skin tests and treating latent TB.
Cytomegalovirus (CMV)	– Viral infection that causes eye disease that can lead to blindness. Symptoms include headache, change in mental status, cough, abdominal cramps,

	diarrhoea, and vision changes such as spots, floaters, or tunnel vision.
Herpes simplex viruses	– Herpes simplex viruses can cause recurrent and painful oral (mouth), anal, or genital ulceration. These are fairly common infections, but if you have HIV, the outbreaks can be much more frequent and more severe.
Candidiasis	– Fungal infection of the mouth (thrush), throat, oesophagus, or vagina. Characterised by white patches on mucous membranes that remain after scraping.
Cerebral toxoplasmosis	– A protozoal infection of the brain that causes neurological symptoms including seizures, altered mentation, and paralysis.

Other Care and Support Services

The needs of women infected with HIV vary depending on the stage of their disease, their home and community situation, and their socioeconomic status. Their needs may be different before and after they deliver, and during breast-feeding. It is critical that PMTCT service providers are aware of care and support services in their localities in order to be responsive and make appropriate referrals. Other care and support services include the following:

- Support groups for mothers have started in some facilities. They provide a mechanism for psychosocial support and ongoing nutrition education for mother.
- Antiretroviral therapy (ART) for those who meet clinical treatment criteria and are able to pay for it.
- Ongoing counselling from PMTCT service providers.
- The TB programme for screening and treatment of latent and active TB as needed. Family planning services available to all HIV-positive women, preferably provided regardless of ability to pay.

— Encourage the women to share experiences and difficulties and help them find solutions. Educate them in hygiene and nutrition and promote a healthy environment and diet for themselves and their families.

— Promote positive interaction with the counselling staff and with one another. Include devotions in the meetings to help meet the spiritual needs of the women, if the group feels that this will be helpful.

— Ask the support group to determine the frequency of their meetings.

— Encourage the women to participate in a micro-enterprise project to obtain loans and start small businesses. Encourage male partners to participate or form their own support groups.

— Organize workshops on topics that are useful to the mothers, including legal matters such as property rights and wills.

— Help HIV-positive mothers or parents with their children to create memory books that document family ties and special events in their family history. Consider including stories, photographs, or mementos in memory books. Through this exercise, mothers are sometimes able to discuss their illness with their older children, while at same time reassuring them that they will be taken care of if she dies. Encourage the women to lobby the government and NGOs to provide better medical care and affordable antiretroviral treatment when it is indicated.

To facilitate mothers' transportation to and from the support group activities, consider reimbursing the cost of transport. Although the cost is low per individual woman, it adds up and may dictate a reduction in the number of group activities. Privacy and space requirements are very challenging. Support groups often meet in improvised or borrowed spaces, which are inappropriate in terms of confidentiality and adequacy of space, ventilation, lighting, etc.

Pregnant mothers are often reluctant to attend, when they are still pregnant. However, these are the mothers who stand to gain the most. Disclosure to partners is still difficult even for this group of motivated, supported women. Some support group mothers die of untreated AIDS in spite of adopting healthy living practices, which is discouraging to the survivors. Many women in support groups have been able to rapidly wean their babies at 3-6 months of age with the help of the education and peer support they have received. Many HIV-positive women have supported HIV prevention activities and some have volunteered to provide community outreach.

UNIVERSAL PRECAUTIONS

As a health care worker (HCW), there will be times when you are exposed to blood and body fluids of patients. These patients could have hepatitis B or C or HIV infections—generally you will not know. Universal precautions are basic good practices that protect you and your patient from the different types of infectious agents in the clinic and hospital, including those carried by patients and staff.

Hand Washing

Hand washing is the single most effective way to prevent the spread of infection in the health care setting and in the home. Hand washing keeps you from transferring contamination from your hands to other areas of your body, to your patients, or to other surfaces you may later contact. Wash hands before putting on gloves and after removing gloves. Wash hands and other skin surfaces immediately and thoroughly, if contaminated with blood or other body fluids. Wash hands between patient contacts.

Standard Precautions

Use barriers to prevent skin and mucous membrane contamination of health care workers, and when contact is made with blood or other body fluids of a patient.

i) Gloves, gowns, masks, protective eyewear, and closed shoes.

   a) Wear latex gloves for touching blood and body fluid, mucous membranes, or nonintact skin of all patients, for handling items or surfaces soiled with blood or body fluids, and for performing venipuncture and other vascular access procedures. Change gloves after contact with every patient. If gloves are reused, adequately disinfect them between uses.

   b) Wear mask and protective eyewear or face shields during procedures that are likely to cause droplets of blood or other fluids, to prevent exposure of mucous membranes of the mouth, nose, and eyes.

   c) Wear gloves, gowns, eye protection or face shields, waterproof aprons, and closed shoes or shoe covers during procedures that are likely to cause splashes of blood or other body fluids.

ii) Decontaminate surfaces with appropriate chemical cleaners after a spill of blood or other body fluids. Ordinary household bleach has five-six per cent chlorine. Prepare a new bleach solution daily and, in addition, whenever the solution becomes cloudy or bloody. If you cannot smell chlorine in the bleach solution, the concentration is no longer strong enough for disinfection.

   a) Use 1:10 bleach solution for disinfecting excreta (eg. bedpans, waste buckets).

   b) Use a 1:100 bleach solution for disinfecting surfaces, medical equipment, patient bedding, and reusable protective clothing before it is laundered; and for rinsing gloves after contact with each patient.

   c) Use 1:100 bleach to clean up spills of blood or body fluids. 70 per cent alcohol does not kill HIV.

iii) Decontamination of instruments and soiled linens.

a) Disinfect soiled instruments in 1:100 bleach for 20 minutes before washing.

b) Soak soiled linen and clothing of infected person in 1:100 bleach for 20 minutes after washing in hot water.

c) When possible, discard latex gloves after use. If they must be reused, rinse soiled gloves, soak in 1:100 bleach for 20 minutes, then rinse again thoroughly and dry on drying racks. They can then be reused for non-sterile procedures, as long as they do not have holes.

iv) Hepatitis B vaccine.

a) Vaccinate all HCWs for hepatitis B, unless they already carry the HBV surface antigen (HbsAg positive) or HBV antibody, indicating previous HBV infection.

MONITORING OF PMTCT PROGRAMME

Continuous internal supervision and monitoring are essential to maintain a quality service provided by a team of providers who feel supported and appreciated. PMTCT services are integrated into busy maternal and child health clinics-often translating to long clinic hours for both mothers and providers. Providers have to assimilate and use new knowledge and skills, some of which challenge their current practices and attitudes.

PMTCT programme supervision is currently provided through regular site visits by a team of supervisors who monitor general services and the laboratory. These visits are undertaken on a monthly basis for well-established services, and more frequently for newer programmes. Supervision and monitoring feed into a more thorough evaluation process, typically provided by an external body.

The objectives of supervising and monitoring are to:

— Improve worker performance by providing support (technical and psychological) and acknowledging their contribution to the success of the programme.
— Obtain valuable information on programme function.
— Facilitate on-site participatory problem-solving.
— Provide workload reports for use in local programme management.
— Assure the programme is successful in meeting the needs of HIV-positive women and their infants and families, in achieving sustainability, and in meeting the reporting requirements that guarantee continued external funding.

Specific activities to assess and discuss:

— Workload, acceptance rate, seropositivity rate, and trends related to these factors. Adherence to protocols (e.g., ANC client flow, HIV testing, sharps disposal, record keeping, and confidentiality).
— Supply and drug management (availability, stock taking, recording, and ordering). These include forms, NVP, HIV test kits, etc.
— Record keeping-accuracy of recording (lab, ANC, maternity, PCR specimens, follow-up), timeliness, interpretation.
— Observation of clinic activities and, with patients' consent, observation of counselling sessions.
— Review of staffing needs and staff training needs.
— Provision of services to referred clients.
— Training needs of staff providing PMTCT services.

Support should be provided through:

— Meeting with team members to provide feedback. If regular team meetings are not feasible, the site supervisor should communicate regularly with his/her staff through other means. Discussing difficult scenarios encountered and sharing experiences among staff.

- Sharing the workload.
- Recognising and addressing stress by providing spiritual and psychosocial support to the staff members who provide PMTCT services. Consider having a chaplain or pastor accompany the supervisory team.
- Training the PMTCT staff on areas needing improvement.
- Conducting regular inventory of HIV test kits, NVP, commercial infant formula, condoms, and other supplies to assure that they don't run out and that they are used to support PMTCT services.
- Reviewing agreed-upon plan to address challenges.
- Establishing job descriptions for staff and conducting performance evaluations.

Supervisors come away with the following:

- PCR specimens.
- Information from registries.
- Completed checklist including the inventory form for HIV tests, NVP, commercial infant formula, and condoms.
- Medications and condoms near or beyond their expiration date.
- A mutually agreed-upon date for return.

After each supervisory support visit, supervisors update the central database and make notes of the specific achievements and challenges at each site. They report actions taken to address the challenges in order to improve services and care where necessary.

Supervision and monitoring provide the insights needed to learn from current PMTCT services and to replicate programmes by applying the lessons learned. It is essential to understand cost, effectiveness, and acceptability.

GLOBAL INITIATIVES TO PREVENT MTCT

HIV/AIDS in children was first recognised in 1983, and it was concluded that vertical transmission of HIV could occur from an HIV-infected mother to her infant during pregnancy and delivery. Two years later, the possibility of HIV transmission through breast-feeding was also acknowledged.

In 1987, the World Health Organisation (WHO) organised a consultation and published a first statement on breast-feeding and HIV, which assessed the limited information available at that time on the risk of HIV transmission through breast-feeding. In 1992, WHO and the United Nations Children's Fund (UNICEF) reviewed new data on breast-feeding and HIV and produced a consensus statement recommending that breast-feeding should remain the standard advice for pregnant women, including those who are known to be infected with HIV, in settings where the primary causes infant deaths are infectious diseases and malnutrition.

In 1997, the Joint United Nations Programme on HIV/AIDS (UNAIDS), UNICEF and WHO issued a revised policy statement on infant feeding and HIV that represented a shift from a population-based policy to one based on a human rights perspective. The statement indicated that women should be empowered to make fully informed decisions about infant feeding and suitably supported in carrying them out. This recommendation, which remains valid, was further clarified during a technical consultation convened by WHO on behalf of its partner United Nations agencies in 2000.

The year 1994 was a turning point, as the results of the Pediatric AIDS Clinical Trials Group (PACTG) protocol 076 demonstrated for the first time the efficacy of zidovudine administered to HIV-infected women throughout pregnancy, labor and delivery and to the newborn for 6 weeks after delivery in reducing vertical HIV transmission by 68 per cent. The ACTG 076 regimen was rapidly introduced as standard practice for reducing the mother-to-child transmission of HIV in western

Europe, Australia and North America but remained too complex and costly to be proposed for use in most developing countries. Research to test the efficacy of shorter and less complex regimens was undertaken in several countries.

In February 1998, the results of a trial of a short course of zidovudine conducted in Thailand were released, bringing new hope that the use of antiretroviral drugs to prevent peripartum transmission of HIV was also feasible in resource-limited settings. The following month, UNAIDS, UNICEF and WHO organised a meeting to review the latest information on interventions for preventing the mother-to-child transmission of HIV and to plan for programme implementation. The decision was taken to implement pilot programmes providing short-course antiretroviral drug regimens and infant feeding counselling and support in several developing countries. Since then, further clinical trials have been conducted, expanding the choice of antiretroviral drug regimens that are safe and effective for preventing HIV transmission to infants in developing country settings.

The meeting of United Nations partners in 1998 showed that mother-to-child transmission of HIV could be reduced most effectively if all available intervention approaches were combined. This led to the definition of a three-pronged strategy comprising:

— primary prevention of HIV infection among parents-to-be;
— preventing unwanted pregnancies among HIV-infected women; and
— preventing transmission from HIV-positive women to their offspring.

The same year, an Interagency Task Team on the Prevention of Mother-to-Child Transmission of HIV was created, comprising the UNAIDS Secretariat, the United Nations Fund for Population Activities (UNFPA), UNICEF and WHO. It was formalised in 1999 by the Coordinating Committee on Health, providing a common platform for action and a clear distribution of roles and responsibilities between the different United Nations agencies for the promotion of the three pronged strategy. In early 2001, the Interagency Task Team was reconfigured to include the World Bank and renamed the Interagency Task Team for the Prevention of HIV in Pregnant Women, Mothers and Infants, to reflect the need to intensify activities for primary prevention among women.

The United Nations General Assembly Special Session on HIV/AIDS (UNGASS) met in June 2001 and set challenging goals for the global fight against HIV/AIDS. The prevention of mother-to-child transmission of HIV featured prominently. The UNGASS Declaration of Commitment on HIV/AIDS includes specific goals for the prevention of HIV infection in infants:

> By 2005, reduce the proportion of infants infected with HIV by 20 per cent, and by 50 per cent by 2010, by ensuring that 80 per cent of pregnant women accessing antenatal care have information, counselling and other HIV-prevention services available to them, increasing the availability of and providing access for HIV-infected women and babies to effective treatment to reduce mother-to-child transmission of HIV, as well as through effective interventions for HIV-infected women, including voluntary and confidential counselling and testing, access to treatment, especially anti-retroviral therapy and, where appropriate, breast-milk substitutes and the provision of a continuum of care. Reaching this goal requires addressing several challenges, developing strong partnerships and raising and allocating substantial resources.

Need of a Comprehensive Strategy

Specific interventions to prevent HIV infection in infants, including the prophylactic use of antiretroviral drugs, have only a limited impact under current programme circumstances. The efficiency of specific programme approaches based on the use of antiretroviral drugs needs to be improved, in particular by increasing client uptake and adherence and by developing and applying more effective regimens. However, the number of HIV-infected women who require the intervention should also be reduced. Only a comprehensive approach that includes primary prevention and reproductive health services for HIV-infected women would lead to the required reductions in HIV infection in infants. This implies significant investment in enhancing health systems to address programme constraints and to effectively deliver a range of interventions to those in need.

All countries have accelerated programme activities in recent years, although progress has been uneven and they are now at various stages of implementation. Thailand and Brazil have made the greatest strides over the years and are seeking to extend services to all pregnant women with HIV. Thailand has now achieved very high levels of coverage of anti-retroviral drug use among HIV-positive pregnant women to prevent HIV transmission to their infants. In Brazil, although coverage is increasing, it varies considerably from one region to another, with a national average of 40 per cent. Ukraine is currently scaling up its programme to the national level. Other countries now plan to rapidly move from demonstration projects to wider implementation.

The organisation of health services and capacity for programme implementation vary between countries, but some common issues arise. In the developing countries, utilisation of antenatal care services is generally high, though in all settings, a varying proportion of women at risk have poor access to antenatal care and HIV/AIDS services, for various reasons. The widespread introduction of voluntary counselling and testing in antenatal care settings has faced many difficulties. Even when voluntary counselling and testing are in place, uptake remains low in many areas. Further, among women agreeing to be tested for HIV, the proportion of those testing positive who receive specific services to prevent transmission to their infants is insufficient, at least in the sites in Africa, which suffer from weak infrastructure and staff capacity. Community support for the programme is often inadequate, and stigma and discrimination remain major barriers to the uptake of services.

The main emphasis in most countries is on providing specific interventions to prevent transmission from HIV-infected pregnant women to their infants, although other programme efforts have been ongoing and programme areas are increasingly being linked. For example, in Thailand, opportunities for strengthening primary prevention are being sought by enhancing HIV prevention services in antenatal and postpartum settings for HIV-negative women and their partners. In Brazil, links are being developed with care, treatment and support programmes for people living with HIV. Most settings, however, still have limited success in increasing the access of HIV-positive women to reproductive health services, including family planning services in the postpartum period.

Political support at the highest level and a sufficient resource base for scaling up seem to be critical to success. Strong partnerships between implementing agencies and links across sectors are also key to ensure the consistency of programme approaches and policy and technical guidelines on difficult issues such as infant feeding in the context of HIV. Vigorous and successful programmes as documented in Thailand and Brazil have benefited from political support at the highest level and have been quick to adapt their strategic approaches in response to research and evaluation data to better meet local conditions, solve implementation problems and innovate in response to new challenges, such as the need to increase access to care for people living with HIV.

REFERENCES

Brahmbhatt H., Kigozi G., Wabwire-Mangen.F, Serwadda D, Sewakambo N et al. "The effects of placental malaria on mother-to-child transmission in Rakai", Uganda. *AIDS* 2003:17:2539-2541.

Global Programme on AIDS. Consensus statement from the WHO/UNICEF consultation on HIV transmission and breastfeeding. *Weekly Epidemiological Record,* 1992, 67:177–179.

Newell M.L., Rogers M. Pregnancy and HIV infection: a European consensus on management. *AIDS* 2002; 16:S1-S18.

UNAIDS, *Children and young people in a world of AIDS*, Geneva, 2001.

______________ *HIV/AIDS and young people: Technical update*, Geneva, 2001.

______________ *Follow-up to the 2001 United Nations General Assembly Special Session on HIV/AIDS. Progress report on the global response to the HIV/AIDS epidemic*, 2003.

USAID, "Efforts to Address the Needs of Children Affected by HIV/AIDS", Washington: The Synergy Project, 2001.

______________ , *The impact of HIV/AIDS on human resources: A literature review*, 2001.

WHO, *Antiretroviral drugs and the prevention of mother-to-child transmission of HIV infection in resource-constrained settings*, 7 January 2004.

______________ , "Strategic approaches to the prevention of HIV infection in infants : report of a WHO meeting". *Morges*, Switzerland, 20-22 March 2002.

______________ *Statement from the Consultation on Breast-feeding/ Breast Milk and Human Immunodeficiency Virus (HIV)*, Geneva 23–25 June 1987. Geneva,1987

WHO/UNAIDS, *Prevention of Mother-to-Child Transmission of HIV: Selection and Use of Nevirapine*, Geneva, 2001.

______________ , *UNAIDS: New Data on the Prevention of Mother-to-Child Transmission of HIV and their Policy Implications*, 2000.

UNAIDS, UNICEF and WHO, *HIV and infant feeding. A policy statement developed collaboratively by UNAIDS, UNICEF and WHO*, Geneva, UNAIDS, 1997

______________ , *Prevention of HIV transmission from mother to child: meeting on planning for programme implementation*. Geneva, 23–24 March 1998.

6

HIV Testing Technologies

The Joint United Nations Programme on HIV/AIDS (UNAIDS) and the World Health Organisation (WHO) recommend the use of second generation HIV surveillance to improve collection, analysis, and use of data essential to AIDS control programmes. The use of second generation HIV surveillance is also promoted to help national and international institutions monitor the epidemic and guide their responses to it. Using second generation HIV surveillance approaches, surveillance systems should be flexible in order to change with a country's needs and state of the epidemic: low-level, concentrated, or generalised.

As countries develop or enhance their surveillance programmes using the principles of second generation HIV surveillance. Second generation HIV surveillance relies on data collected from biological surveillance (serosurveillance), behavioural surveillance, and other sources to describe a country's HIV epidemic and respond effectively. HIV serosurveillance data are used to estimate HIV prevalence rates and geographic distribution of infection, monitor trends over time in specific population groups, and identify subpopulations at increased risk for infection.

As biological surveillance is the primary method for determining HIV prevalence rates locally or nationally, accurate HIV testing is critical for second generation HIV surveillance. With advances in diagnostic immunology, HIV testing technologies have improved greatly.

The only way to decide whether or not somebody is infected with HIV is to have him/her take an HIV test. The role of the laboratory in this programme is primarily that of determining the serostatus of consenting prenatal clients, their spouses, and the babies born to seropositive mothers.

ENZYME IMMUNOASSAYS (EIAS) TESTS

Enzyme immunoassays (EIAs) are more accurate than earlier generations of EIAs, and the latest generation of HIV rapid tests can provide results similar to EIAs in less than 45 minutes with minimal experience and no equipment. These rapid tests enable testing for HIV surveillance activities in areas where testing could not previously occur and for hard-to-reach populations (e.g., female sex workers) who may not be accessible through clinical services.

WHO recommended, HIV testing strategies are based on HIV prevalence rates, and existing HIV testing technologies used for biological surveillance. They also include information regarding strategies and technologies for use in diagnostic testing since data from diagnostic testing may also be used as a source of surveillance information. They outline methods for selecting and evaluating testing technologies appropriate to a country's epidemic state and needs. Since accurate results are important in biological surveillance for HIV, quality assurance measures are also addressed.

HIV testing can be conducted for surveillance, diagnosis, or blood screening. In developing countries, most HIV testing for surveillance purposes is conducted as part of sero-prevalence surveys among population groups such as women attending antenatal clinics, patients with sexually transmitted infections, female sex workers, or injection drug users. In addition, the results of testing for diagnostic purposes and for blood screening purposes, as well as results of regular testing of other groups, can provide additional prevalence data for surveillance purposes.

RAPID HIV ANTIBODY TESTS

While ELISA and Western blot HIV tests have been the most widely used diagnostic tests for HIV, are considered to be the most accurate, and are frequently used as confirmatory tests, they are not readily available and are expensive. It is preferable to use rapid HIV antibody tests for the following reasons:

- The tests produce results quickly, usually in five to 30 minutes.
- The use of rapid HIV tests increases the number of persons who learn their HIV status.
- It reduces the follow-up efforts necessary to locate and counsel HIV-positive persons who do not return, because results are given the same day.
- A rapid HIV test is the only real option for a woman who presents late in pregnancy or early in labour.
- Technically, rapid tests are easier and more feasible to implement at health centre level, where there are no highly qualified laboratory staff and sophisticated equipment.
- A rapid HIV test gives two possible results: positive or negative. This simplifies interpretation by the provider.

A rapid test for HIV detects antibodies in a person's blood due to infection with the virus. It does not detect the virus itself. With antibody tests there are two circumstances in which the result may not be a true indication of the presence or absence of infection as follows:

- It usually takes six weeks to three months or sometimes as long as six months after infection by the HIV virus for seroconversion to take place. During this "window period," HIV antibody tests are negative, even though the person is infected.

— Newborns may acquire maternal HIV antibodies through the placenta without necessarily picking up the HIV virus itself. Maternal antibodies may persist in the baby's blood until 12-15 months of age. During that period the baby tests positive even though it is not infected.

Testing Procedure

i) Enter the necessary information about the client in the register.

ii) Collect 2 cc of whole blood from venipuncture for all the prenatal tests or perform a finger prick to obtain necessary blood.

iii) Perform a Determine HIV rapid test as the first test on all clients who consent. In primary health centers where there are no laboratories, Oraquick is substituted as the first test, since it can use saliva from an oral swab instead of blood.

iv) If the first test is negative, perform no confirmatory tests the same day. The results of our pilot study indicate that the sensitivity of Determine was 98.5 per cent and specificity was 97.5 per cent. The Oraquick test on saliva also has high sensitivity and specificity.

v) If the first test is positive, perform a second test (Hema-Strip, Oraquick, HIV spot, HIV check or Capillus). If discrepant results occur, perform a third tiebreaker rapid test and consider collecting a specimen for confirmatory testing by ELISA and Western blot testing.

vi) The laboratory staff will deliver the prenatal test results to the counsellor.

POLYMERASE CHAIN REACTION (PCR) TEST

If polymerase chain reaction (PCR) testing is available, collect blot specimens only from babies of seropositive mothers at six weeks after delivery. Send them for the PCR test, which identifies the HIV virus itself and therefore indicates true infection in the baby. In contrast, the detection of HIV antibodies in newborns may not necessarily indicate infection, because they may be acquired transplacentally from the mother.

— Assure that the blood specimens entirely fill each of the five circles of the blot card and soak all the way through the filter paper.
— Dry all loaded blot cards for three hours or more at room temperature; place them in individual paper envelopes without a desiccant and store in a clean dry place at room temperature. For shipping or hand carrying specimens from outlying facilities to a central lab, place the individual plain paper envelopes in one or two of the Tyvek plastic bags with desiccants. When the specimens arrive at the central lab, remove them from the Tyvek plastic bags and store them in individual paper envelopes without a desiccant in a clean dry place at room temperature until final processing or until shipping to a reference lab.
— For shipment to the reference lab, collect all blot specimens and put them in a large Tyvek bag with desiccant.
— Remember to apply biosafety practices: wear gloves and keep the work environment clean and disinfected before and after work.

APPROACHES OF HIV TESTING

The selection of HIV testing approaches for serosurveillance depends on contextual factors, such as country policies and, given the epidemic state, appropriate population groups and settings for HIV testing. Unlinked anonymous HIV testing is only conducted in clinic settings where blood is collected regularly for other purposes. If feasible, such testing should be conducted in settings where referrals to voluntary counselling and testing are provided.

Linked testing with informed consent is the preferred approach when the specimens are collected solely for HIV testing, for example, HIV surveillance in populations not accessible through clinic settings. When specimens are collected solely for HIV testing, unlinked anonymous testing with informed consent may also be used, depending on the country's relevant policies and guidelines.

A code should be assigned to every specimen tested for HIV. The code is used to identify each specimen during testing procedures. It is unique to a specimen, and it may or may not be linked to personal identifying information, depending on whether the HIV testing is linked or unlinked. The code can be linked to demographic and risk behaviour information (in linked testing) that is obtained at the time the specimen is collected.

Unlinked anonymous testing without informed consent is only conducted in clinical settings in which a specimen of blood originally collected for other purposes, such as syphilis testing at antenatal clinics, is tested for HIV after all information that could identify the source of the blood is removed from the specimen. Thus, the test result may not be traced back to the patient nor may he or she be informed of the test results.

To ensure patient anonymity at the clinic and laboratory, one staff member should collect the specimen and a different staff member should perform testing. One staff member (clinician or laboratory technician) should collect and process the specimen for routine clinical testing and for unlinked anonymous HIV testing. The processing of the specimen for unlinked anonymous HIV testing requires removing an aliquot of blood and placing it into a new tube that is labelled with a new code not linked to any personal identifying information. Another staff member should perform unlinked anonymous HIV testing. In some settings, one staff member (the laboratory technician) is responsible for both collecting the specimen and performing unlinked anonymous HIV testing.

In these situations, it is suggested that another staff member process the specimen for unlinked anonymous testing (i.e., remove an aliquot of blood and place it in a new tube labelled with a new code not linked to any personal identifying information). At the time of specimen collection, a staff member collects demographic information and medical history from the patient. This information is recorded onto a clinic form along with the code on the specimen. After the specimen is processed for unlinked anonymous HIV testing and the aliquot is labelled with a new code, the same staff member records the new code onto a surveillance form and abstracts the needed demographic information onto the form.

The unlinked anonymous HIV test results can then be matched with the demographic information for analysis by the new code. It is important that the anonymity of the specimen not be compromised by the collection of too much demographic information that may allow identification of individuals. In settings where blood is not routinely collected for other purposes, unlinked anonymous testing without informed consent is considered unethical. Therefore, in these situations, linked testing with free access to voluntary counselling and testing should be provided, or, if country policy permits, unlinked anonymous testing with informed consent should be conducted.

In unlinked anonymous testing with informed consent, the participant is asked whether he or she would agree to participate in the HIV surveillance study and informed that the results of the HIV test performed will be unlinked by removing all personal identifying information from the specimen. Therefore, it will not be possible to trace which participants have positive test results. The participant should be provided free access to HIV testing and counselling. The person can refuse to participate in the study, thereby introducing a possible participation bias.

Linked testing involves linking the results of the HIV test with the person tested and allows the person to receive his or her HIV test results. This method requires obtaining informed consent and providing pretest and post-test counselling. Linked testing may or may not occur in a clinical setting. Linked testing can be either confidential or anonymous. Since the person tested may receive the test results, linked testing requires additional confirmatory HIV testing. In linked confidential testing, a person agrees to have an HIV test with the assurance that the test result will be kept confidential and only selected health-care providers may be informed. HIV test results can be matched to the person by a code linked to personal identifying information.

For linked confidential testing, a staff member obtains informed consent and provides pretest counselling prior to specimen collection. The specimen is then labelled with a code that can be linked to personal identifying information. After linked confidential HIV testing is performed, the test results are given to the person, along with post-test counselling. In linked anonymous testing, a person consents to having an HIV test. The methods for collecting and processing the specimen are the same as for linked confidential testing. However, the specimen is labelled with a code not linked to any personal identifying information, and only the person can link himself or herself to the test result.

Sero-surveillance is typically conducted in large clinics, outpatient clinics at hospitals, or health centers. Countries with concentrated epidemics or low-level epidemics focus primarily on specific population groups who are perceived to be at high risk for infection, for example, female sex workers and their clients, injection drug users, or men who have sex with men. Therefore, venues attended by such persons are selected as sentinel sites; these may include clinics that treat sexually transmitted infections, drug treatment centers, correctional facilities, brothels, bars, and clubs.

The recent modification of a type of HIV test termed "detuned assay" or Standardised Testing Algorithm for Recent HIV Seroconversion (STARHS) is now available only as a research tool for measuring HIV incidence. Its use in non-research settings has not been approved in any country. STARHS allows for determining whether an HIV-infected person has been recently infected. Specifically, it indicates whether the person has seroconverted (produced HIV antibodies) within an average of about 130 days prior to being tested. This ability to distinguish recent from older infections permits estimation of recent HIV incidence based on a single cross-sectional survey. Such estimates of HIV incidence can be extremely valuable for evaluating the current trends of HIV infection.

Many types of specimens can be used with HIV testing technologies for HIV biological surveillance:

i) whole blood,
ii) plasma,
iii) serum,
iv) oral fluids, and
v) urine.

The choice of specimen collected depends on logistics, populations and sites selected, and the HIV testing strategy. Specimens must be collected, tested, and stored in an appropriate manner in order to obtain accurate and reliable results. For serosurveillance activities, specimens are usually collected and stored prior to HIV testing at a regional or national laboratory. Serum, plasma, and dried blood spots can be stored and tested at a later date; specifications for storage will depend on the type of specimen collected.

Specimens not tested on site at the local level will need to be transported to a regional or national laboratory for testing. The methods by which specimens are transported will depend on the country's infrastructure. Few countries may have courier systems linking health-care facilities and laboratories. More frequently, the field surveillance staff members themselves transport the specimens from the local to the national laboratory.

Whole blood, serum, and plasma, which can be collected by venipuncture or finger stick, have the following advantages in HIV testing:

i) Have higher concentrations of HIV antibodies than urine or oral fluids.
ii) Have potential for additional routine testing (e.g., syphilis, hepatitis B, hepatitis C) from a single specimen.
iii) Have potential for special studies
iv) Are easy to collect and test in clinical settings with a laboratory and a trained phlebotomist.
v) Are easy to collect in non-clinical settings (whole blood from finger stick).

The following are the disadvantages:

i) Require invasive collection technique.
ii) Require skilled technician (for collecting and processing serum or plasma).
iii) Compared with urine and oral fluids, require more equipment (e.g., needles, tubes, or lancets) and biohazard waste facilities.
iv) Is difficult to collect serum or plasma in non-clinical settings if venipuncture is required.
v) Compared with oral fluids, pose a greater risk to health-care workers and technicians through inadvertent exposure, both because of higher antibody concentrations and the use of sharp collecting devices.

Other specimens besides blood and blood products can be used for HIV testing. For linked testing, where informed consent must be obtained, oral fluids may be used. Urine is the only other specimen (besides blood) routinely collected at some clinics where unlinked anonymous testing could be conducted. The following are the advantages in HIV testing:

i) Do not require a trained technician for specimen collection and processing.

ii) Do not require contact with possibly contaminated laboratory materials, e.g., used needles or lancets that need biohazard waste facilities.

iii) Oral fluids can be collected in a variety of field settings, including non-clinical settings.

iv) Oral fluid collection may be more acceptable to hard-to-reach populations than specimen collection requiring venipuncture or finger stick. Therefore, a greater percentage of the target population may agree to be tested.

The following are the disadvantages in HIV testing:

i) Urine EIA tests are less sensitive and specific than blood-based tests.

ii) Urine specimens must be tested at a laboratory (EIA); no rapid test is currently available.

iii) Oral fluid collection may require special equipment.

iv) Currently available testing technologies for use with these specimens are limited.

v) Are likely to cost more than using serum or plasma.

vi) May require an additional specimen (e.g., blood) for confirmation.

vii) Cannot be used to perform additional testing for special studies.

Blood needed for an HIV test can be collected either by venipuncture (whole blood, serum, plasma) or by finger stick (whole blood). To collect blood by venipuncture, follow local clinical or laboratory procedures. The following steps are recommended for processing blood collected by venipuncture:

i) *Step 1*: Collect up to 10 ml of blood from the patient's vein into a sterile 10 ml tube. For serum, blood is collected in a red-top tube (without anticoagulants). For plasma, blood is collected in a purple-top tube (with anticoagulants, e.g., EDTA). For safety reasons, the use of an evacuated blood collection system (e.g., Vacutainer tube) is recommended. If the blood specimen will not or cannot be processed immediately, collect the blood in a purple-top tube with EDTA. Let the blood stand for at least 20-30 minutes, and then remove plasma carefully with a pipette so as not to get too many red blood cells. Process and test within 24 hours to avoid hemolysis of the specimen. A dried blood spot can also be prepared at this time using anti-coagulated blood.

ii) *Step 2*: Centrifuge the specimen to separate the serum (without EDTA) or plasma (with EDTA). If blood is collected for serum, allow the blood to stand for at least 20-30 minutes so that a clot will form before centrifuging. In general, the specimen should be centrifuged at 300-400 g or 1,200 to 1,500 RPM for 10 minutes.

iii) *Step 3*: After the specimen is centrifuged or has had time to separate, use a clean pipette (do not pour) to remove an aliquot of 0.5 to 2.0 ml off the top layer. Transfer it to another sterile labelled tube (plastic, not glass) or cryovial and tighten the cap. The specimen is ready for storage and testing.

To store serum and plasma, consider the following:

i) Make sure the cap is tight on the labelled cryovial or plastic tube. Place the cryovials in a cardboard freezer box with a partitioned insert.

ii) If the specimens are to be transported to the testing laboratory, immediately pack the box upright in a cooler containing cold packs to produce an ambient temperature of 4°C within the cooler. If cold packs are not available, serum specimens can remain at room temperature for up to three days. Longer periods at room temperature may result in bacterial over-growth and breakdown of the specimen.

iii) If specimens are held at the collection site for longer than three days prior to shipment to the laboratory where testing will be performed, freeze specimens at -20° C in a nonfrost-free freezer. For long-term storage, specimens should ideally be frozen at -70°C in a non-frost-free freezer.

iv) Limit the number of freeze/thaw cycles to five because multiple thaws will affect antibody levels and therefore test results.

Blood collected by finger stick can be used to perform a rapid test or make a dried blood spot on filter paper. A dried blood spot may be preferred in rural settings and nonclinical settings, which often do not have trained phlebotomists and laboratory facilities with appropriate equipment (e.g., centrifuges):

i) To obtain a finger-stick specimen, massage the finger (preferably the middle or ring finger), which will cause blood to accumulate at the tip of the finger.

ii) Cleanse the finger pad with 70 per cent isopropyl alcohol. Wipe away alcohol with sterile gauze pad.

iii) Use a sterile lancet to firmly prick the finger pad. Wipe the first drop of blood off the finger with sterile gauze before collecting subsequent blood to place on the rapid test apparatus or on the filter paper for the dried blood spot.

If the original puncture is inadequate, the same site should not be reused; another site or finger should be used. Avoid milking or squeezing the puncture as this may cause hemolysis of the specimen and could invalidate the test result. The earlobe may be pricked instead of the finger. Blood from a finger or earlobe stick can be used to make dried blood spots. Although finger stick is the most typical method, dried blood spots can also be obtained by using blood collected in a tube with an anticoagulant. Dried blood spots have the advantage of being easily transported, without the need for a cold chain.

i) Apply blood directly from a finger or a pipette onto special filter paper. The paper may come with preprinted circles that will contain approximately 100L blood when completely filled. If the paper does not have preprinted circles, place blood on the paper so that it makes a circle with a 1.5 cm diameter. Allow the blood to soak through and fill the entire circle.

ii) Label the side of the filter paper with a code after the filter paper is saturated with blood (circle is filled).

iii) Suspend filter paper strips containing the filled circles during the drying process to allow air to circulate around the paper. Stands for holding the strips are commercially available. However, strips may also be dried by placing them between two books (taping the edges of the strips to the books with sticky tape) on a table or a laboratory bench top so that the blood-containing part of the paper is not in contact with the surface of the table or laboratory bench top. Be sure not to get tape on the blood spot.

iv) Let the blood spots air dry at room temperature for at least 4 hours. Do not heat or stack blood spots, and do not allow them to touch other surfaces while they are drying.

v) After blood spots have been adequately dried, wrap the strip in one sheet of glassine paper or plastic to prevent carryover of specimen from one sheet to another.

vi) Place the wrapped strips in a gas-impermeable bag with desiccant and humidity indicator cards. Approximately 20 strips may be placed in each bag. Bags may be kept at room temperature for up to 30 days and then stored at 4° C for up to 90 days. If the dried blood spots in their plastic bags are to be stored longer than 90 days, they should be maintained at -20° C. Properly stored dried blood spots have been shown to be stable for at least two years. The bags should be placed in a sturdy envelope for shipment.

A variety of EIA protocols exist for using urine specimens; however, no rapid tests are available at this time for use with urine specimens. A few important considerations when collecting urine are:

i) A minimum of 200 L of urine is usually required for use with a urine-based EIA test kit.
ii) Specimen can be collected at any time of day and need not be midstream.
iii) A preservative may be added to the specimen for storage, although it is not required.

Oral fluids can be used with both modified EIAs and rapid tests. Rapid tests using oral fluids are currently under field evaluation. The following general steps to collect a specimen are provided:

i) Use a specially treated absorbent pad attached to a plastic stick (usually provided by the test kit manufacturer).
ii) Place the pad in the person's mouth against the inner cheek for the length of time specified in the manufacturer's instructions. Then place the pad into a vial containing a preservative solution.

Due to the test complexity, oral fluid specimens collected for EIAs are sent to a national laboratory for analysis. Urine specimens should be placed in plastic cryovials containing a preservative. Urine specimens with a preservative may be stored up to one year at 4°-8° C. Urine specimens for HIV testing must not be frozen. Oral fluid specimens can be stored from 4° to 37° C for a maximum of 21 days. Oral specimens should be refrigerated during shipment. Specimens can be frozen (-20° C) for a limited time. Once thawed, they can be refrozen once. Consult the test kit insert prior to testing for more specific storage information.

The plastic tube, cryovial, or filter paper containing the specimen must be labelled with a code at the time of collection and processing. If labels are used, make sure the label is placed on the side of the tube, not on the cap. Preprinted cryolabels designed to adhere during freezer storage should be used when specimens are stored in cryovials. Surveillance coordinators should provide the field staff responsible for specimen collection with a series of labels or permanent markers and the codes to be used.

For unlinked anonymous testing, label the tube only with a new code unlinked to personal identifying information. A separate laboratory logbook or line listing for surveillance activities should be maintained to record HIV test results by the corresponding code. The logbook should be accessible only to laboratory and surveillance staff; it should be secured in a locked drawer or cabinet when not in use to ensure the confidentiality of the persons' test results as well as their participation in surveillance activities.

For unlinked anonymous testing, the logbook or line listing should contain only the new codes and corresponding HIV test results; no personal identifying information on the patients whose specimens are tested should be included. HIV test results can be matched by the new code to the demographic information abstracted earlier on the surveillance form.

HIV testing technologies can currently identify:

i) Antibodies to HIV (e.g., EIA, rapid test, Western blot, immuno-fluorescence assay, particle agglutination)
ii) Specific HIV antigens (e.g., EIA, antigen testing)

iii) HIV viral nucleic acid (e.g., by polymerase chain reaction or other techniques)

iv) HIV (by viral culture)

For surveillance as well as diagnostic purposes in developing countries, technologies that identify HIV antigen, viral nucleic acid, or HIV itself are expensive, technically more difficult, and more often affected by laboratory error. In most industrialised countries, current diagnostic testing procedures use an EIA to screen a specimen, and if it is reactive, the result is confirmed by testing the specimen with a Western blot. In addition, compared with Western blots, EIAs and rapid tests are less expensive, do not require as high a level of technical expertise to perform and interpret, and produce fewer indeterminate results.

ACCESS TO HIV TESTING AND COUNSELLING: CHALLENGES AHEAD

Knowledge of HIV status has always had the potential for benefiting an individual's health and wellbeing and for helping to prevent the further transmission of HIV. Knowledge of HIV status has been especially beneficial when it has enabled people to access care, support and treatment, in the form of psychosocial support; home-based care; nutritional support; palliative care; treatment for opportunistic infections, tuberculosis and sexually transmitted infections; and antiretroviral therapy.

However, in many places, access to care, support and treatment has been very limited. Access to antiretroviral therapy has been, and still is, largely unavailable for most of the people needing it. Three million people needing antiretroviral therapy are envisaged to have access to it by the end of 2005. Further, in many communities, people who are HIV positive, or fear they are, face stigma and discrimination.

Denial, lack of access to care and treatment as well as stigma and discrimination have acted, and continue to act in some places, as serious disincentives to people wanting to know, or to disclose, their HIV status. In this context, HIV testing has had a problematic place in the response to the epidemic, especially in the early years of the epidemic. Some policy-makers have promoted mandatory testing for either the general population or for certain groups considered to be at "high risk". This has been promoted largely as a means of identifying people who might pose a risk of transmitting infection to other people. When carried out, such testing has often had a punitive outcome (such as discrimination, stigma, imprisonment and/or loss of employment) and no health benefit.

From a public health viewpoint, there has been concern that mandatory testing tended to drive away the very people who needed HIV interventions. Mandatory HIV testing has been rejected as being neither feasible nor affordable, as being ineffective in achieving public health objectives and as being an impermissible violation of human rights. For these reasons, the World Health Assembly, WHO, UNAIDS, the United Nations Commission on Human Rights and many other international and national groups have spoken out against mandatory testing.

HIV testing has also been problematic in the context of clinical care. This is because, in many places, HIV testing has reportedly either not been conducted at all as part of clinical care or has been conducted without consent, confidentiality, counselling, the provision of results or any follow-up care to benefit health. Even in places where people with AIDS occupy more than 50 per cent of hospital beds, almost none of these people have been diagnosed as HIV positive or told that they have AIDS.

Although this phenomenon may result from fear that these patients will face discrimination or be denied health insurance, etc., if they are diagnosed as having AIDS, it also appears to be a form of medical denial that ultimately does not serve the best interests of these people or their families or communities. Few protocols have been developed to provide guidance about the appropriate use of HIV testing in clinical care settings.

Neverthless, voluntary HIV counselling and testing (VCT) has functioned as an effective and ethical public health tool. In the standard model of VCT, the overall objective has been prevention, with an emphasis on confidentiality and voluntary individual decisionmaking, including protecting the individual's decision not to be tested and/or not to learn the result of the test. Counselling in VCT has involved dialogue between counsellor and client, emphasised safe behaviour, provided support for behavioural change and been neutral or even dissuasive in respect of the client's decision to be tested.

Since it has been confidential and has been non-threatening with regard to testing, VCT has tended to attract those who might otherwise shy away from HIV intervention. From a public health perspective, VCT has therefore served to connect many people to paths related to HIV prevention and care. This model of VCT has been shown to be effective in increasing understanding of risks, providing a supportive environment in which to learn one's HIV status, achieving behavioural change for prevention and increasing access to support. When it has been widely implemented in a context of community mobilisation, it has also helped to open up the epidemic; decrease denial, stigma and discrimination; increase opportunities for counselling for couples; and involve greater numbers in the response.

However, VCT has not been implemented on a large scale in many low-income communities and countries, including those hardest hit by the epidemic. One reason is that the standard model of VCT is expensive and difficult to implement, as it requires substantial infrastructure, time and trained staff. Another reason is the fact that the uptake of VCT has been low where there are disincentives to learning of one's status.

Denial, stigma and discrimination as well as lack of access to treatment, care and support continue to exist in many countries and communities. Testing without consent, confidentiality or beneficial outcomes still remains a major problem in many places. Trying to address these realities is important in implementing any HIV testing and counselling programmeme or procedure.

Nevertheless, important developments in the political, social and care contexts of the epidemic compel the implementation of different, innovative and expanded approaches to HIV testing and counselling while remaining committed to the principles of voluntariness, informed consent and confidentiality.

The United Nations General Assembly Special Session on HIV/AIDS held in 2001 and other important political initiatives provide evidence that, in the last few years, the international community, many governments and key elements in the private sector have overcome denial and are demonstrating a new commitment to addressing the prevention and care challenges of the epidemic.

There has also been recognition of the real extent of the resources needed to fight the epidemic, and new efforts have been made to mobilise these, such as the World Bank Multi-Country HIV/AIDS Programme for the Africa Region and the Global Fund to Fight AIDS, Tuberculosis and Malaria. Further, political leadership, community involvement and multisectoral approaches have shown that stigma, denial and discrimination can be overcome and positive results can be reached in prevention and care.

In addition to this new political and social context, access to treatment and care, which has always been an ethical and human rights imperative, has now become much more of a real possibility. The prices of critical treatments, including antiretroviral drugs, have dropped drastically, creating the opportunity for millions more to benefit from life-saving treatment and, in the case of infants of HIV-infected mothers, to benefit from preventing transmission from mother to child.

Governments have shown much greater commitment to increasing access to treatment, care and support and, indeed, formalised this commitment at the United Nations General Assembly Special Session on HIV/AIDS. They have also agreed to reduce by 20 per cent the proportion of HIV infections in infants by the year 2005 by providing HIV testing and counselling services to the majority of pregnant women in affected countries.

At the XIV International AIDS Conference in Barcelona in July 2002, a global target of antiretroviral treatment for 3 million people by the end of 2005 was accepted as the immediate goal for increasing access to treatment. Several national and international initiatives to increase access to treatment are currently under way, including the formation of the International HIV Treatment Access Coalition and various partnerships involving governments and pharmaceutical companies and the companies and initiatives involved in the generic production of antiretroviral agents.

Numerous programmes have been started and significant funding identified for preventing mother-to-child transmission of HIV and providing treatment and support to mothers and their infants, partners and families. The vital role of people living with HIV/AIDS in prevention and care has been increasingly recognised and made a reality.

Given this evidence of an international and national movement toward greater access to treatment and care, HIV testing and counselling has a critical role in this process. As knowledge of positive infection status is a prerequisite to the provision of antiretroviral drugs, including in preventing infection from mothers to their infants, HIV testing and counselling becomes a necessary and first step in realising greater access to treatment.

Even where treatment is not available, knowledge of HIV status, and hence HIV testing, can be critical in preventing HIV infection from being acquired and transmitted; can help to reduce stigma and discrimination; and can act as an essential diagnostic tool that leads to better management of a person's health. Nevertheless, the vast majority of people in the world do not have access to HIV testing and counselling by which to learn of their HIV status and, with this knowledge, to access prevention, care and treatment services that are available now or are likely to become available in the future.

According to some estimates a global total of 180 million people would need HIV testing and counselling annually by 2005. This includes: up to 100 million in preventing mother-to-child transmission, 12 million in clinical care and 67 million in prevention. These figures are daunting, but they represent the potential number of those in need of testing and counselling and not necessarily the pool of people who would actually avail themselves of such services. Further, successes in other public health endeavours give hope that achieving something close to these goals is possible.

Another immense challenge is the potential cost of HIV testing and counselling services. Assuming a modest cost of US$ 10 per client for 180 million clients, this would result in a global annual cost of US$ 1.80 billion. Given this extremely high cost, urgent needs include being strategic, lowering the cost of counselling and testing through the use of different appropriate models while maintaining quality and setting priorities among efforts in terms of populations served and the objectives to be reached. Among other things, costs could be reduced by reducing the time spent in pre-test and post-test counselling. The costs would probably vary according to setting.

Other major challenges are the lack of human, technical and financial capacity to increase access to HIV testing and counselling. In terms of human capacity, there is the need for: sufficient numbers of counsellors from various backgrounds; sufficient time for counselling appropriate to various settings; and sufficient numbers of phlebotomists and laboratory staff.

Strategies to address these needs include greater use of people living with HIV/AIDS as both lay and professional counsellors, using community volunteers in counselling and educational processes and creating a new cadre of paid counsellors, thereby recognising (non-nurse) counsellors as a professional category. Employment of such counsellors would be less expensive and allow greater potential for expansion. Appropriate eligibility criteria and appropriate curricula and training would be required for these counsellors.

In terms of technical capacity, physicians, nurses and other health care providers need training in: the ethical principles of informed consent, confidentiality, ethical disclosure and partner counselling; storage and quality management of test kits; the use of test kits, including rapid tests; and record-keeping.

Another major challenge, the level of which differs according to local circumstances, involves the environment in which HIV testing and counselling are delivered. HIV testing and counselling programmes need to be tailored to the realities faced by potential clients, including : the prevalence of HIV infection; the actual availability of treatment and care; the existence of denial, discrimination and stigma; and barriers to testing and counselling posed by age, legality, socioeconomic status and gender. Among other things, these factors significantly affect the likelihood that a client will access services, agree to be tested, return to receive testing results and remain in the programme to receive the necessary follow-up.

The lack of appropriate policy, legal and enforcement frameworks are important obstacles to ensuring the ethical and effective implementation of HIV testing and counselling. Women face obstacles in many societies in which their unequal status prevents them from being able to exercise real autonomy throughout the process of testing, counselling and follow-up. There are legal barriers to consent for minors and barriers caused by the criminalisation of sex work and drug use. Models of implementation should be tailored to address these elements.

HIV testing and counselling should always be implemented in a manner sensitive to the community context, especially such factors as denial of or lack of access to services; coercion; lack of understanding, consent and confidentiality; and punitive or negative outcomes around testing. Every effort should be made to ensure that testing and counselling is voluntary, ethical and conducted in a supportive environment, results in beneficial outcomes and is conducted in a legal context enabling redress by the individuals concerned when ethical principles have been unjustifiably violated. These challenges should be incorporated in finding new and creative ways to overcome the challenges of scaling up and ensuring wider access to testing and counselling rather than continuing to inhibit the HIV testing and counselling process itself. Such an approach is especially indicated, given the positive changes in the HIV prevention and care context noted above and the crucial importance of HIV testing and counselling to prevention, treatment and care at this stage of the epidemic.

VCT model of HIV Testing and Counselling

In the context of HIV testing and counselling for preventing HIV infection, the VCT model was developed in the mid-1980s as the standard of care for individuals seeking to know their infection status. This model places as much, if not more, emphasis on counselling as on testing. Counselling in this model is usually one-to-one, is client-centred and focuses on providing HIV-related information, helping clients to develop a risk reduction plan and exploring whether the client wishes to be tested. The sequence followed is : pre-test counselling, HIV testing (if voluntarily chosen) and post-test counselling.

For those who test negative, post-test counselling might include further risk-reduction counselling and support. For those who test positive, post-test counselling might include psychosocial support and referral to necessary medical services and social support services. Post-test services might also include support and crisis management, provision of condoms, partner notification and/or testing, and referral to sexually transmitted infection services.

Informed consent is usually not problematic in the standard VCT model of HIV testing and counselling. The client initiates the use of the services and participates in pre-test counselling, which involves a discussion about the choice to be tested. However, there have been cases in which those participating in VCT have been pressured to do so, such as women or adolescent girls pressured by partners or employees pressured by employers. In some jurisdictions, minors cannot give consent to be tested and are thus legally barred from accessing VCT on their own. Those under the age of consent need to overcome legal barriers to the uptake of VCT.

VCT in many places has fulfilled a vital need, has helped to mobilise communities around HIV/AIDS and has reduced denial and stigma surrounding HIV/AIDS. Where it has functioned well, it has usually benefited from a supportive policy and legal environment and community mobilisation to increase uptake. However, some problems are associated with the standard VCT model of HIV testing and counselling.

This model requires a great deal of time and infrastructure and a well-supported staff of trained counsellors. This makes it costly, slow and difficult to scale up quickly where the demand for HIV testing and counselling is high or growing. Strict adherence to in-depth pre-test counselling and an emphasis on secrecy may make this model too intense and complicated for some who wish to undergo an HIV test on a more routine basis.

The efficacy and cost-effectiveness of the different elements of this model of VCT have not been fully established. For instance, in some settings and with some groups, counselling alone may be sufficient to change behaviour, such as for young people or for those to whom providing testing services is difficult, such as truck drivers. For other settings or groups, one-on-one counselling may be too intensive and costly compared with some sort of group, structural or environmental process that may lead to behavioural change.

Operational research is needed to explore a variety of models for delivering VCT for prevention purposes. VCT services are not necessarily reaching those who need them, such as young people or vulnerable groups. Nor are such VCT services sufficiently linked to care services, especially for these groups. In some places, special approaches are necessary to improve access to VCT and to overcome legal, social and cultural barriers experienced by young people, women and others, such as sex workers, mobile populations, migrants, injecting drug users, prisoners and rural populations. Successful approaches have taken the form of outreach, mobile clinics, youth-specific clinics, integration of VCT into family planning or other service packages, such as VCT along with harm-reduction programmes for drug users. Links with other vital services can be the incentive by which to involve some hard-to-reach groups in a more holistic service package.

Supportive Environment to HIV Testing and Counselling

The widespread use of HIV testing and counselling has been largely avoided in the past, as individuals or communities decided that the potential benefits of knowing HIV status did not outweigh the potential harms, such as stigma and discrimination. However, some communities, determined to face the epidemic openly and strongly, have been able to encourage more widespread knowledge of HIV status by maximising the benefits that could be made available to those who know their status and providing encouragement and social support to undergo testing and counselling. In these communities, a supportive environment, more widespread knowledge of status and providing care and support at whatever level available have turned the tide on denial, stigma and discrimination.

Now, when knowing HIV status may result in even greater benefits, communities, governments, donors, non-governmental organisations and others should more aggressively make the link between HIV testing and counselling and health care, psychological and social support and treatment. Given the serious consequences of a positive HIV test result, those considering being tested for HIV should always be supported. Further, where stigma, discrimination and lack of care and treatment still exist, much greater efforts have to be undertaken to create a supportive environment. Such an environment is essential to encourage those who need or want HIV testing and counselling to be willing and able to take it up. The three main elements of a supportive environment that would help to attract clients to health care or VCT services, support them to consent to a test and receive the result and enable them to follow through with the relevant interventions that would enhance their health and their lives are: strong links to treatment, care and support; community mobilisation; and an appropriate policy and legal framework.

Links to treatment, care and support: HIV testing and counselling should only be conducted to enhance the health and well-being of the client. In this regard, it should always be linked to the provision of care and support, and where possible, treatment. Not only is this linkage ethical, it can also create dynamics that galvanise prevention and care efforts and greatly support their effectiveness. Knowledge of HIV status has always had the potential to increase the ability of an individual and his or her health care provider to enhance health and well-being. Unfortunately, millions of people have missed this opportunity in the course of the epidemic, as they have grown ill and died without any knowledge of their status. Even in resource-constrained settings where care and treatment are very limited, every effort should be made to link knowledge of status with available benefits. These might include: prevention of onward transmission to partners; better diet and nutrition; initiatives for positive living; home-based care; access to therapy for opportunistic infections, tuberculosis and sexually transmitted infections; palliative care; planning for the future; and post-test social support, such as that found in post-test clubs and other community groups.

There are important new opportunities to provide treatment to millions who need it. From the outset, efforts to increase access to HIV testing and counselling should be linked to the growing number of initiatives and programmes designed to increase access to antiretroviral therapy, management of tuberculosis, treatment for sexually transmitted infections and interventions to prevent transmission to women and children. Since knowledge of HIV status is a prerequisite to antiretroviral treatment and to the prevention of mother to child transmission, HIV testing and counselling forms an essential component of these initiatives and programmes.

Community mobilisation: Community mobilisation is critical to the success of increasing access to and uptake of HIV testing and counselling. It can be used to overcome the barriers of ignorance, denial, stigma and discrimination and to encourage people to utilise HIV testing and counselling services. Awareness of HIV/AIDS, which has largely been achieved, is not the same as understanding it and being motivated to do something about it. Community mobilisation can be the force that gets people to act on their knowledge.

There are powerful examples of communities supporting their members to enter and follow through with HIV testing and counselling services. This has occurred in communities defined by geography and in those defined by membership in a particular group, such as young people, women, sex workers, truck drivers and migrants. In fact, peer support is often the trigger for individuals to take up testing and counselling. Community mobilisation efforts that have been successful involve such elements as : political leadership; community-based media and social marketing campaigns; community discussion forums; using community role models, including people living with HIV/AIDS; integrating HIV testing and counselling into existing community services or into the activities of existing community groups (men, women and young people); community campaigns and social marketing against stigma and discrimination; training community health care and other service providers in nondiscrimination and ethics; and community faith-based initiatives.

Despite all the recognition and rhetoric concerning the increased involvement of people living with HIV/AIDS, they continue to be a tremendously underutilised resource. Involving people living with HIV/AIDS is not tokenism but is instead essential to achieving a holistic understanding of and response to the epidemic and is also practical and effective. With appropriate support, people living with HIV/AIDS can be engaged in almost all aspects of HIV testing and counselling: in designing, managing and administering programmes; as professional and lay counsellors; as people who help to provide psychosocial support; as links to other services and resources; and as people who help to mobilise the community through advocacy and activism around HIV testing and counselling.

Policy and legal framework: Appropriate legal and policy frameworks are important in combating discrimination based on HIV status. Many countries need legislation that recognises discrimination based on health status, including HIV/AIDS, and provides legal sanctions for it. Such legislation should cover both the public and private sectors. In many places, the legal system is weak and people do not have access to the courts. However, even in such places, much can be accomplished if there is legal support for those aggrieved and a few key court cases on HIV-related discrimination are brought to trial and won.

Policy and practices that encourage non-discriminatory behaviour are important. Policies against HIV-related discrimination and favouring support should be implemented in all places that provide government services, including uniformed services and social services, such as public health, housing and public assistance. Much can and should be done in the private sector.

The workplace remains a key area for policies that protect workers against discrimination and help to provide them access to prevention and care services, including HIV testing and counselling. Other areas should be made more supportive of HIV testing and counselling. One example is the counterproductive policies of some insurance companies to deny benefits once HIV/AIDS is diagnosed. Not only does such a policy result in a tragic denial of support, but it also makes clinicians less likely to diagnose HIV, document it in clinical records and provide appropriate follow-up.

In many places, health care workers continue to discriminate against those living with HIV/AIDS. They do this partly because they lack sufficient training about HIV and AIDS and partly because of a valid fear of acquiring HIV infection through their work. If the offer of HIV testing and counselling is to become standard practice where clinically indicated, health care workers should be empowered to provide health care in an ethical and nondiscriminatory manner. Such empowerment would involve:

a) working in the context of an appropriate policy framework;
b) training in the management of HIV and the use of universal precautions;
c) providing the means by which to implement universal precautions and post-exposure prophylaxis, where antiretroviral drugs are available; and
d) training in the principles of informed consent and confidentiality, nondiscrimination, acceptance and compassion.

Many models of HIV testing and counselling are being implemented in various countries and communities. Some of these are effective and should be scaled up; others are unethical, do not lead to health benefits and can traumatise and disable those tested. Examples of best practices regarding HIV testing and counselling models urgently need to be documented and disseminated. Any scaling up of HIV testing and counselling in the circumstances outlined above should lead to general improvement in the medical ethics and efficacy surrounding current practice relating to HIV and any other conditions where informed consent, confidentiality, counselling and testing are at issue.

In Brasil, the country's policy and practice of universal access to antiretroviral agents provide a vitally important context for the HIV testing and counselling that is implemented on a wide scale there. In this regard, Brazil is a showcase for a country's ability to purchase, manufacture and distribute antiretroviral therapy in resource-constrained settings. It is also a model in which to study the positively reinforcing and dynamic interrelationship between prevention, care and treatment. With almost universal access to treatment and a concomitant decrease in denial, stigma and discrimination, HIV testing and counselling has become a standard and essential part of prevention and care efforts.

Experience in Brazil also demonstrates how HIV testing, in terms of regional and national infrastructure for testing, must be scaled up if prevention and care are to be carried out effectively. The overall costs of provision of testing, counselling and antiretroviral therapy have been recouped in terms of lower hospital care costs and the reduction of other social and economic losses arising from the illness and death of those living with HIV/AIDS.

Zambia represents a model of rapid expansion of VCT services, having gone from a few such services in non-governmental organisation and research sites in 1999 to some 100 sites nationwide in 2002. Each of Zambia's 73 districts now has at least one testing and counselling facility, and 185, 892 clients have been tested and counselled. By 2004, the target is that at least 25 per cent of sexually active Zambians will know their serostatus. Important lessons have been learned on the need for political commitment, the efficiency and costs of different models, the reasons for uptake and dropout, the effectiveness of referrals to other services, the involvement of community partners and operational challenges related to logistics, supplies and quality assurance.

In Zimbabwe, a high-prevalence country, community surveys indicated that 50-70 per cent of adults believed themselves to be infected even though most were not. At the same time, about 90 per cent were not aware of their actual HIV status. This combination of perception and reality resulted in little incentive to change behaviour. As the provision of HIV testing was very uneven across the country, an initiative to increase access to VCT was begun. Because public surveys indicated that people considered an HIV test to represent a new start in their lives, the initiative was called New Start. Under this initiative, VCT has been provided in public clinics, in AIDS service organisations, in private company clinics, in freestanding clinics and in outreach programmes. Research has shown that social marketing of the programme has been successful in increasing access and uptake as well as in decreasing stigma and discrimination. The performance of different models has been evaluated, and lessons have been learned from each model. These lessons will guide future efforts to scale up.

REFERENCES

Centers for Disease Control, "Perspectives in disease prevention and health promotion update: Universal precautions for prevention of transmission of human immunodeficiency virus, hepatitis B virus, and other pathogens in health-care settings", *MMWR Morb Mortal Wkly* Rep 1988; 37(24): 377-88.

Downing R.G., Otten, R.A., Marum E., et al.. "Optimising the delivery of HIV counselling and testing services", *J Acquir Immune Defic Syndr Hum Retrovirol,* 1998; 18(4): 384-8.

Janssen, R.S., Satten, G.A., Stramer, S.L., Rawal, B.D., O'Brien, T.R., Weiblen, B.J., et al, "New testing strategy to detect early HIV-1 infection for use in incidence estimates and for clinical and prevention purposes", *JAMA* 1998; 280: 42-8.

Martinez, P.M., Torres, A.R., Oritz de Lejarazu, R., Montoya A., Martin, J.F., Eiros J.M., "Human immunodeficiency virus antibody testing by enzyme-linked fluorescent and Western blot assays using serum, gingival-crevicular transudate, and urine samples", *J Clin Microbiol,* 1999;37(4):1100-6.

National Committee for Clinical Laboratory Standards, "Procedures and devices for the collection of diagnostic blood specimens by skin puncture", *NCCLS document H4-A4,* 1999.

National Committee for Clinical Laboratory Standards, "Procedures for the handling and process of blood specimens; Approved guidelines", *NCCLS document,* H 18-A. 1990.

Respess, R.A., Rayfield, M.A., Dondero, T.J., "Laboratory testing and rapid HIV assays: applications for HIV surveillance in hard-to-reach populations", *AIDS* 2001; 15 (suppl 3):S49-S59.

Richmond J., and McKinney, R. , (ed.), *Biosafety in microbiological and biomedical laboratories*, Washington (DC):U.S. Government Printing Office; 1993.

Rose N.R., Conway de Macario E., Folds J.D., Lane H.C., Nakamura R.M., editors. *Manual of clinical laboratory immunology*. 5th ed. Washington (DC): ASM Press; 1997.

Stetler H.C., Granade T.C., Nunez C.A., Meza R, Terrell S., Amador L., et al. Field evaluation of rapid HIV serologic tests for screening and confirming HIV-1 infection in Honduras. *AIDS* 1997;11:369-75.

Tam, M.R., "Serological and biomolecular detection of human immunodeficiency virus types 1 and 2", Seattle (WA): *Programme for Appropriate Technology in Health (PATH)*. June 1999.

UNAIDS, *HIV Testing Methods: UNAIDS Technical Update*, (UNAIDS Best Practice Collection Technical Update). Geneva: UNAIDS, November 1997.

______________ , *Voluntary Counselling and Testing: Technical update*, Geneva, 2000.

______________, *The Impact of Voluntary Counselling and Testing: A global review of the benefits and challenges*. Geneva, 2001.

UNAIDS/WHO , *Guidelines for second generation HIV surveillance*, Geneva: UNAIDS/WHO. WHO/ CDS/CSR/EDC/2000.

______________ , Operational characteristics of commercially available assays to determine antibodies to HIV-1 and/or HIV-2 in human sera", *Report* 11. January 1999. Geneva: UNAIDS/WHO.

______________ , "UNAIDS/WHO Recommendations. The importance of simple/rapid assays in HIV testing", *Weekly Epidemiological Record*. 1998; 73:321-28.

______________ , *Guidelines for organising national external quality assurance schemes for HIV serological testing*, UNAIDS/96.6 Geneva: UNAIDS/WHO; January 1996.

WHO, *Biosafety guidelines for diagnostic and research laboratories working with HIV*, Geneva: 1991. *WHO AIDS Series* 9.

World Health Organisation and Joint United Nations Programme on HIV/AIDS, *Guidelines for Using HIV Testing Technologies in Surveillance: Selection, Evaluation, and Implementation*. 2001.

WHO/GPA., *Statement from the consultation on testing and counselling for HIV infection*, Géneva 16-18 November 1992.

7

HIV/AIDS and its Momentum

The worldwide struggle against HIV/AIDS has intensified in the past few years. The political momentum to tackle AIDS has grown. Public opinion in many countries has been mobilised by the media, non-governmental organisations, activists, doctors, economists, and people living with HIV/AIDS. Communities and nations are progressively taking the lead in responding to the epidemic with increased political commitment, resources and institutional initiatives. But this new political resolve is not universal. An unacceptable number of governments and civil society institutions are still in a state of denial about the HIV/AIDS epidemic, and are failing to act to prevent its further spread or alleviate its impact.

By failing to act, governments and civil society are turning their backs on the possibility of success against AIDS. Where the moment of action has been seized, there is mounting evidence of inroads being made against the epidemic. Alongside the familiar achievements of Senegal, Thailand and Uganda, there are new successes on every continent. Despite emerging from genocide and conflict, Cambodia responded to the threat of HIV in the mid-1990s and has achieved marked declines in both the levels of HIV and the high-risk behaviours associated with its transmission. The infection rate among pregnant women in Cambodia declined by almost a third between 1997 and 2000. The Philippines has acted early to forestall the epidemic, keeping HIV rates low with strong prevention efforts and the mobilisation of community and business organisations.

Brazil remains a leading example of the integration of comprehensive care and a renewed commitment to prevention. The numbers of new HIV infections have been kept much lower than forecast less than a decade ago, while the 1996 decision to establish a legal right to free medication has brought treatment and care to more than 100 000 HIV-positive people. As a result, the number of annual AIDS deaths in Brazil in 2000 was a third of that in 1996. In Africa, Zambia's focus on HIV prevention among youth and its efforts to involve businesses, farmers, schools and religious groups in the fight against AIDS are proving successful.

Examples of success come both from settings where HIV prevalence is low and from those where the impact of HIV/AIDS is already substantial. Both environments present challenges. Even where rapid increases in the epidemic are evident, yet population-wide prevalence is low, it is all too easy to marginalise HIV. In heavily affected countries, the challenge has been that of building the political conviction that solutions are possible in the face of the overwhelming impact of the epidemic.

GLOBAL PRIORITIES

The new political momentum culminated in June 2001 when the membership of the United Nations met in a Special Session of the General Assembly to agree on a comprehensive and coordinated global response to the AIDS crisis. The members adopted a powerful Declaration of Commitment, and reaffirmed the pledge (made by world leaders in their Millennium Declaration) to halt and begin to reverse the spread of AIDS by 2015.

The UN General Assembly Special Session on HIV/AIDS differed from the hundreds of meetings and summits held on AIDS in the past 20 years in this crucial respect: it was a meeting of all States, acting as governments. As such, it yielded both a common mandate and a basis for political accountability.

The Special Session's Declaration of Commitment, adopted unanimously, now serves as a benchmark for global action. Its targets and goals include the need to:

- secure more resources to fight AIDS, increasing annual spending to US$7–10 billion in low- and middle-income countries;
- ensure, by 2005, that a wide range of prevention programmes are available in all countries;
- by 2005, to ensure that at least 90 per cent of young people aged 15–24 have access to information, education and services necessary to develop the life skills needed to reduce their vulnerability to HIV, and 95 per cent by 2010;
- reduce by 25 per cent the rate of HIV infection among young people aged 15–24 in the most affected countries by 2005 and globally by 2010;
- reduce by 20 per cent by 2005 and 50 per cent by 2010 the proportion of infants born with HIV;
- by 2003, enact or strengthen anti-discrimination and human rights protections for people living with HIV/AIDS and for vulnerable groups;
- by 2003, develop or strengthen participatory programmes to protect the health of those most affected by HIV/AIDS;
- empower women as an essential part of reducing vulnerability to HIV;
- by 2003, develop national strategies to strengthen health-care systems and address factors affecting the provision of HIV-related drugs, including affordability and pricing; and
- make treatment and care for people with HIV/AIDS as fundamental to the AIDS response as is prevention.

Underpinning the renewed global resolve in tackling AIDS is a series of shifts in fundamental thinking about the epidemic.

Firstly, we now realise that the HIV/AIDS epidemic is at an early stage of development and that its long-term evolution is still unclear. Despite the epidemic's manifest potential for explosive growth within a matter of years, its overall dynamic needs to be considered in a timeframe of decades.

Secondly, successful, proven approaches to HIV prevention have been identified, and the need for a particular emphasis on young people has been recognised. In every country where HIV transmission has been reduced, it has been among young people (and with their determination) that the most spectacular reductions have occurred.

Thirdly, community mobilisation is the core strategy on which success against HIV has been built. Fostering such mobilisation requires eliminating stigma, developing partnerships between social and government actors, and systematically involving communities and individuals infected and affected by HIV/AIDS.

Fourthly, access to comprehensive care and treatment for HIV/AIDS is not an optional luxury in global responses. Access to care is a basic necessity in programming in every setting—from the wealthiest to the poorest —and needs to encompass the full continuum, including home-based and palliative care, treatment of opportunistic infections and anti-retroviral therapy.

Responding to demands for more equitable access to care is integral to creating broad, demand-driven strategies that respond to the desire by households and communities to protect themselves from HIV and its effects. Demand-driven HIV prevention is likely to succeed far more readily than supply-driven approaches.

Fifthly, addressing the economic, political, social and cultural factors that render individuals and communities vulnerable to HIV/AIDS is crucial to a sustainable and expanded international response.

The Millennium Development Goals, arising from the UN Millennium Summit of September 2000, include a commitment to halt and begin to reverse the global spread of AIDS by 2015. They also include the following goals: to halve global poverty; ensure primary school education for all; promote gender equality and empower women; and reduce child mortality while improving maternal health. This total package is integral to success in alleviating the impact of AIDS.

Finally, lack of capacity to absorb increased resources allocated for HIV/AIDS, while posing challenges, is no reason to delay the boosting responses in countries expressing commitment to an expanded response. Assessments of programme readiness carried out by UNAIDS, together with rapid responses to calls for proposals from the new Global Fund to Fight AIDS, Tuberculosis and Malaria, are both demonstrations of immediate and substantial unmet needs in AIDS programming in much of the world.

INTERNATIONAL RESPONSES

Growing political engagement in the response to AIDS is grounded in two decades of AIDS activism, led by individuals and communities whose lives have been touched by the epidemic. Organisations as diverse as the Gay Men's Health Crisis in New York, The AIDS Support Organisation in Uganda, the Save Your Generation Association in Ethiopia, Grupo Pela Vidda in Rio de Janeiro, and many hundreds of others like them, are built on the same foundations: an initially small group of people responding to the impact of AIDS by coming together to provide mutual support and take action.

An activist movement responding to AIDS now exists globally. It has many aspects: community groups providing home-based care, treatment activists working through media and the law courts to extend access to HIV drugs, networks such as the International Council of AIDS Service Organisations and its regional bodies, and associations of HIV-positive people nationally and internationally, together with positive women's networks.

The presence of non-governmental and community-based organisations was notable at the United Nations General Assembly Special Session on HIV/AIDS in June 2001, providing a sense of urgency and conscience to Member State deliberations. The Global Fund to Fight AIDS, Tuberculosis and Malaria has modelled a new way of working by including on its Board not only non-governmental organisation representatives but also a seat for people who are themselves directly affected.

The bedrock of activism, sustained in communities motivated to take action against AIDS, is key in driving political momentum locally, nationally and globally. From within the United Nations, Secretary-General Kofi Annan has helped catalyse growing global engagement. In April 2001, at the African Summit on HIV/AIDS, Tuberculosis and Other Related Infectious Diseases, in Abuja, Nigeria, he issued a global call to action in the fight against AIDS. The personal priority he has given to AIDS has helped energise the United Nations system, as well as engage political and business leaders in the challenge.

At the Millennium Summit of the United Nations in September 2000, 43 Heads of State and Government, from both countries heavily affected and those less so, referred to AIDS as one of the most pressing problems worldwide. Presidents and prime ministers, particularly those from Africa and the Caribbean, but also those in Asia and Western and Eastern Europe, are displaying a personal commitment to the fight against AIDS. Support for expanded AIDS responses has been voiced by religious leaders and groups of all faiths—from Catholic and Protestant bishops and the Patriarch of All Russia, to associations of Imams and networks of Buddhist monks in South-East Asia.

AIDS is now a prominent issue at international gatherings—North and South. It has been on the agenda of summits and decision-making forums of the G8 and G77 nations, the Organisation of American States, the Organisation of African Unity, the Commonwealth of Nations, the European Union, the Association of South-East Asian Nations, and the Caribbean Community Secretariat (CARICOM). Both the World Economic Forum and the World Social Forum (in Porto Alegre) have held key sessions on AIDS and its global implications. The UN Security Council held its first-ever debate on AIDS in January 2000—the first time it had examined a health or development issue. Since then, it has held two more public debates on AIDS.

Partnerships are emerging in response to AIDS, with increased involvement across the whole of government as well as between governments, civil society and the business sector. Trade unions and women's and youth organisations are engaging in AIDS-related activities, often for the first time. Business coalitions on AIDS have spread, especially in Asia and Africa. Globally, businesses have recognised the need for a proactive AIDS agenda, and efforts in this direction are being spearheaded by the Global Business Council on AIDS.

The International Labour Organisation (ILO) became UNAIDS' eighth Cosponsor in 2001. It has engineered a new code of conduct designed to protect and support workers with HIV/AIDS and to use workplaces more effectively in the fight against AIDS. Meanwhile, philanthropic foundations, such as the Bill and Melinda Gates Foundation, are making increasingly imaginative and generous contributions —both financial and intellectual—in prevention, in supporting care access, in reducing mother-to-child transmission, and in the search for a vaccine, among others.

Emergency responses, whether to conflict or disaster, are beginning to deal with AIDS more effectively in emergency settings, be they refugee camps or war-torn zones. The World Food Programme is lending its support to AIDS responses in its field of operations, while the International Federation of Red Cross and Red Crescent Societies has begun to tackle AIDS-related stigma, starting with its workers and volunteers.

The new paradigm in access to care is beginning to take effect, and long-standing global inequities are being challenged. From disputes before the World Trade Organisation, to court cases in South Africa, debate in relation to essential medicines has been resolved in favour of lowering trade barriers to access. The principle of preferential pricing for HIV drugs for low- and middle-income countries has been largely accepted in the pharmaceutical industry. Prices have begun to drop and countries' rights to invoke compulsory or voluntary licensing arrangements on patented drugs and medications were affirmed clearly at the World Trade Organisation meeting in Doha, Qatar, in late 2001. Generic versions of many antiretroviral drugs now exist. The World Health Organisation has begun a process of quality assessment of HIV medicines (brand-name and generic) and is widely publishing the results in order to promote the rational use of drugs as well as affordable prices.

Important progress has been made in the prevention of mother-to-child transmission. New guidelines on anti-retroviral therapy and infant-feeding for HIV-infected mothers have been developed. Manufacturer Boehringer Ingelheim's offer, in July 2001, of free nevirapine for low- and middle-income countries is gradually being taken up. But this also means that voluntary counselling and testing need to go beyond the 1 per cent of women in sub-Saharan Africa currently being reached. Antenatal care infrastructure has to expand. And safe infant-feeding by HIV-infected mothers must become an actual choice, rather than a theoretical one. Much work remains to be done, however, in transforming the successes of small pilot projects into large-scale programmes. As with the epidemic in general, access to HIV treatment also has governance and security dimensions. Even in the poorest countries, in urban areas, in particular, there is already a huge backlog in demand for HIV treatment. If treatment remains inaccessible, or if it is only extended to small elites, social tension might be further inflamed. Already, AIDS 'miracle cures' have given rise to local instability in India, Nigeria, Thailand and elsewhere.

Funding for HIV/AIDS

Aggregate spending for HIV/AIDS in 2002 was projected to approach US$3 billion in low- and middle-income countries, much of it underwritten by international assistance. In the most heavily affected region (sub-Saharan Africa), international spending on HIV/AIDS has risen well above the US$165 million figure documented in 1998—a trend projected to continue in 2002. In the past few years, domestic spending on HIV/AIDS has also increased significantly in many countries.

The mismatch between need and funding is one of the biggest obstacles to controlling the epidemic. Most poor countries still struggle to boost their spending, even to levels that fall far short of the need. If current budgetary trends continue, donor support in 2003 will still be much less than the bare minimum required for basic prevention and care programmes. Despite the fact that millions of people living with AIDS are being impoverished even further by the epidemic, many of them have to pay for their own care. It is a virtual certainty that out-of-pocket spending accounts for a considerable share of overall AIDS spending everywhere, especially among the poor.

Among the few prominent exceptions is Brazil, where out-of-pocket HIV/AIDS spending is a low 6 per cent, thanks to strong public funding. By contrast, private, out-of-pocket spending in Rwanda, for example, accounted for 93 per cent of total HIV/AIDS spending in 1998–1999, and only 7 per cent came from government and donors. Such high dependence on out-of-pocket spending, particularly when it is the poor who are paying, is of grave concern. It is imperative that new ways be found to reduce the share of total AIDS spending by the poor. One way is to boost support to public health care and other social services, as part of broader, poverty-focused programming.

A detailed calculation of the estimated total financial need in low- and middle-income countries for HIV/AIDS, done by an international team convened by the UNAIDS Secretariat, has shown that, in 2005, US$9.2 billion will be required. That amount is several times greater than the spending projections for 2002 in low- and middle-income countries. A sustained increase therefore has to be achieved, with annual spending rising progressively to an annual total of US$9.2 billion in 2005. Of that amount, US$5.4 billion is required for countries with a gross domestic product of less than US$2000 per person. This projected, staggered rise in spending assumes that many countries cannot immediately mount the entire range of activities needed. Indeed, most countries would take several years to build up the human and infrastructural capacity to programme their expanded responses. These projections are based on conservative estimates of possible costs for each of the 18 prevention, treatment and care services used in the calculations of overall resource needs, and do not include costs for building up infrastructure. If expenditures on AIDS were to remain at current levels, the funding shortfall would grow to at least US$7 billion by 2005, unless significant amounts of additional funding become available.

It is estimated that, overall, between one-third and one-half of the required funding could come from domestic private and public sources. Certainly, national ownership and responsibility are vital ingredients for effective AIDS responses, and the list of countries that devote significant funds towards combating the epidemic has grown considerably in recent years. In addition, the Abuja Declaration, adopted at the Organisation of African Unity's special summit on AIDS in 2001, included a pledge that 15 per cent of national budgets would be allocated to health spending. This would require a significant increase in spending for several countries. But many of the worst-affected countries rank among the poorest in the world, and are unable to finance their entire HIV/AIDS efforts domestically. National AIDS programme managers, health directors and health ministers from 14 sub-Saharan African countries in 2001 pinpointed the funding gaps their countries faced. In each of six of the countries (Kenya, Lesotho, Malawi, the United Republic of Tanzania, Uganda and Zimbabwe), the gaps ranged from US$50 million to US$200 million. Measured against the countries' limited tax bases and low income levels, the shortfalls highlight the need for greater donor assistance. Up to 80 per cent of total resources needed in sub-Saharan Africa and South and South-East Asia will have to come from international sources. This funding shortfall cannot be met from a single source. Several distinct sectors are involved in responding to AIDS, each of which has its own comparative advantages.

International donors account for approximately two-thirds of budgeted HIV/AIDS spending in 2002 in low- and middle-income countries, the bulk of it in the form of Official Development Assistance. In addition to providing funding, many donor countries can also draw on domestic technical resources and help build solidarity directly between their own communities at home and those in the recipient countries.

Multilateral organisations represent another important channel of assistance. They are well placed to ensure that internationally accepted scientific and technical standards are applied, to help promote consensus on the effective approaches, and to help AIDS programmes achieve longer-term financial sustainability. Agencies such as UNDP, UNFPA and UNICEF, for example, are also important channels for deploying funding from bilateral donors in countries where they lack programming capacity.

A range of major international foundations have substantially increased their support for population activities—from US$99.3 million in 1995 to an estimated US$539 million in 2000. Many of the activities relate to sexual education, condom provision and other HIV/AIDS-related programmes. The Bill and Melinda Gates, Rockefeller, Ford, Marie Stopes, Kaiser, and United Nations Foundations, and the Open Society Institute, among others, are all active in international HIV/AIDS programming. The newest funding channel is the Global Fund to Fight AIDS, Tuberculosis and Malaria. Its comparative advantage is the ability to rapidly direct new resources towards programmes that hold the best chances of success, in the countries with the greatest need.

Global Fund to Fight AIDS, Tuberculosis and Malaria

Operating since January 2002, the Global Fund to fight AIDS, Tuberculosis and Malaria was set up as a financial instrument to complement existing funding for programmes addressing HIV/AIDS, tuberculosis and malaria. The Fund concentrates on generating additional resources and making them available at the community and country levels.

As a public-private partnership, the Fund's Board includes official country representatives, as well as representation from the business sector, non-governmental organisations and communities directly affected by the epidemic. The UNAIDS Secretariat, together with two of its Cosponsors, are nonvoting members of the Board. The Fund coordinates its activities with governments, civil society, non-governmental organisations, UNAIDS, the private sector, and donor agencies.

Total pledges to the Fund stood at just under US$2 billion in April 2002. Most of the pledged funds came from the Official Development Assistance budgets of donor countries, and from the endowments of major philanthropic organisations. In its first grants, announced in the same month, the Fund committed more than US$616 million over two years to support programmes in over 30 countries to combat AIDS, tuberculosis and malaria. Around 60 per cent of these funds will support HIV/AIDS prevention and treatment programmes, and most of these grants specifically include funding to purchase antiretroviral treatment. A further 15 per cent of funds will go to programmes to fight AIDS, together with malaria and/or tuberculosis.

Multi-Country HIV/ AIDS Program for Africa

Managed by the World Bank, the Multi-Country HIV/AIDS Programme for Africa came into effect in 2001. The Programme takes the form of large, sero-interest loans to support governments over several years—loans that are largely channelled as grants to communities and civil society organisations. The emphasis is on increasing access to HIV/AIDS prevention, care, support and treatment programmes (with an emphasis on vulnerable groups), as well as mitigating the impact of the epidemic. Financed to the tune of US$500 million, the first stage was approved by the World Bank in September 2001, and is now supporting 13 countries in sub-Saharan Africa. In February 2002, the Bank provided US$500 million more, which is expected to support another 12–15 countries. In addition to country programmes, it is intended to support subregional and cross-border initiatives—for example, those targeting major transport routes such as the Abidjan-Lagos Corridor. A similar initiative is now also under way in the Caribbeans. Totalling US$155 million, the Multi-Country HIV/AIDS Prevention and Control Project for the Caribbean works as a five-year loan programme that allows countries to obtain separate loans or credits to finance their national HIV/AIDS prevention and control projects.

Debt relief

Reducing the debt burdens of poor countries also has the potential of boosting the AIDS response where it is most needed. The debts of the 38 highly indebted poor countries (HIPC) amount, on average, to more than four times their annual export earnings. These debt burdens mean that annual debt-servicing obligations can undermine countries' social spending, including that required for their HIV/AIDS and orphans responses.

In 16 African countries in 2001, governments were still spending more on servicing debts than on the health of their citizens. The HIPC debt initiative, devised by the World Bank and International Monetary Fund, is one attempt to relax those constraints and enable countries to allocate more resources to social development. Under the initiative, eligible countries qualify for debt relief if they meet certain conditions, including the adoption of economic adjustments and the drafting of poverty-reduction strategies in which social spending is given priority. Applicant countries are encouraged to include HIV/AIDS programmes in these strategies. UNAIDS and its Cosponsors are working to provide technical and other support to help countries integrate HIV/AIDS into poverty reduction strategies.

Although only a few countries had completed the entire HIPC process by early 2002, 24 countries had reached the first of the two stages in this debt-relief process (the so-called 'decision point'), putting them in line for debt reduction. In those cases, debt relief could free significant sums of money for spending on public health care.

Initial indications are that, on average, HIPCs will spend about 25 per cent of their annual interim debt relief on health care. As for AIDS, data from 10 low-income African countries from this group suggest that, together, they were budgeting some US$32 million for AIDS activities, or about 5 per cent of their HIPC savings, in 2001.

The UNAIDS Secretariat has reviewed the first generation of 25 full and interim Poverty-Reduction Strategy Papers prepared by sub-Saharan African countries to gauge how well they were dealing with HIV/AIDS. The review was based on four criteria: analysis of the relationship between AIDS and poverty has been carried out; the main strategies from the country's national AIDS plan feature in the poverty reduction strategy papers; medium-term AIDS prevention and care goals and indicators for monitoring poverty are used; and short-term initiatives to fight HIV/AIDS have been incorporated. In some other HIPC countries, however, little or no money from debt-relief proceeds has been specifically allocated to HIV/AIDS. In addition, this source of funding is not available to several low- and middle-income countries that are experiencing severe HIV/AIDS epidemics.

Role of Business Sector

The business sector also has an important role to play in funding an expanded response. Approximately 7 per cent of the total resource need is for workplace prevention programmes, which private enterprises can fund. The scale and range of business involvement in the fight against AIDS are growing, but they are still only a fraction of their potential. Showing the way, meanwhile, are AIDS-related business initiatives that capitalise on key business strengths. For example, UNAIDS is working with MTV to help bring awareness to teenagers around the world. In Asia, the Thai Business Council has teamed up with the Thai Red Cross and other partners to integrate HIV/AIDS into the standard curricula taught to merchant sailors in maritime colleges. Debswana, in Botswana, has introduced prevention, treatment and care services for its employees and their spouses, effectively reducing HIV incidence, especially among its youngest workers.

NATIONAL RESPONSES

Today all most all counties have recognised that AIDS is not just a health issue; it is fundamental to development, progress and security. Now, presidents and prime ministers throughout Africa, the Americas, the Caribbean, Asia and Eastern Europe are publicly displaying personal commitment to the fight against AIDS. This high-level political commitment has acquired more than symbolic weight. In country after country, rapid advances have been made when presidents and prime ministers took control of the AIDS response, often chairing the national coordinating bodies dedicated to dealing with the epidemic. But the symbolic value of stirring declarations of commitment is also important, for it sounds the alarm, helps spur people to action, and generates hope among those who might have felt marginalised by a disease few talked about publicly.

Governments' Role

Involvement of people living with HIV

AIDS is crucial if the barriers of stigma, discrimination and denial are to be overcome. But if they are to choose candour over secrecy, people living with the virus need to have an environment that protects them. For this to happen, leaders have to safeguard fundamental human rights. This may mean reviewing and improving legal instruments, and extending people's access to legal services and information. In the Philippines, for example, the 1997 National AIDS Law was developed in consultation with a wide range of stakeholders by the Ministry of Justice. More recently, the Indian Ocean Partnership explicitly affirmed the need to respect human rights in order for the HIV/AIDS strategies to succeed.

The commitment of countries' top political leaders must cascade across all levels of government. In that vein, the May 2001 Annual Meeting of Francophone Parliamentarians drafted a framework document to guide West African legislatures on making effective contributions to national responses. On the other side of the continent, in mid-2001, 80 members of parliament in the United Republic of Tanzania created the Tanzanian Parliamentarians AIDS Coalition, to advocate inside and outside of parliament.

Political leadership at a more local level is also important. In Belarus, the National HIV Council has counterparts at the regional and municipal levels. Each is assured political clout by the fact that a deputy head of local government chairs the local councils. Already, some of these decentralised HIV councils are helping place HIV on local agendas.

Mobilising all sectors of society

An important role for governments is to clear the way so all sectors of society can contribute to the response. Countries that have employed multisectoral approaches have seen their national response bolstered by the involvement of religious, cultural and community groups or associations, employers, trade unions and non-governmental organisations. In Africa, especially, it has become commonplace to include multiple ministries, as well as representatives of civil society and other development partners in high-level political coordination structures. Togo provided a recent example when its president set up and chaired a National AIDS Council that now includes representatives from several government ministries, civil society and the private sector. This kind of example is being repeated in other countries. In the Caribbean, for example, the Government of St Kitts and Nevis recently expanded its National AIDS Advisory Committee to include trade unions, non-governmental organisations, organisations of persons living with HIV/AIDS, religious organisations, and the private sector.

The fact that more and more national AIDS councils, commissions or similar bodies are led by presidents, prime ministers and vice-presidents reflects the threat posed by AIDS to national development. This high-level leadership not only demonstrates political commitment, but also increases the pressure on non-health ministries to develop activities to fight AIDS within their normal programmes.

Political mobilisation and policy-making bodies must be managed carefully to avoid creating confusion between existing institutions that already implement AIDS-related activities. Ministries of Health, for example, have traditionally taken the lead on AIDS programming, often through National AIDS Control Programmes. One way to avoid possible conflicts is by setting clear responsibilities for coordination, advocacy and policy-making in a manner that does not undermine the mandate of health ministries or of other existing structures.

In Kenya, for example, the National AIDS Control Council takes the lead on coordination and evaluation of all activities against AIDS, while the Ministry of Health still manages the mainly health-related interventions. Large-scale assistance efforts, such as the World Bank's Multi-Country AIDS Program for Africa, have provided funds to both the National AIDS Control Council as well as to the Ministry of Health.

Within such coordinated frameworks, more and more countries are showing how individual ministries can integrate AIDS into their existing mandates, often in coordination with other ministries and agencies. In Sri Lanka, for example, the Ministry of Labour, the Health Education Bureau, and the Ministry of Women's Affairs have taken on the issue of sexually transmitted infections and HIV/AIDS in free-trade zones. As a result of these zones' attraction for both national and international migrant workers and changing income structures, the risk of HIV/AIDS can be increased in these zones and surrounding areas.

The ministries cooperate with non-governmental organisations to provide prevention services for workers in the zones. And, in the transport sector, the Ministries of Railroads in China and Mongolia have launched programmes for young migrant workers travelling in their respective countries.

Since AIDS is an issue that concerns society as a whole, responses to the epidemic must be linked to national development issues and to development instruments such as Poverty-Reduction Strategy Papers. In Africa, for example, 10 countries have budgeted about 5 per cent of their debt savings for AIDS activities under the highly indebted poor countries (HIPC) debt-relief programme.

Meanwhile, Thailand's Eighth National Economic and Social Development Plan, which factors AIDS into the nation's overall development strategy, treats AIDS as inseparable from other development problems. This reflects the Plan's focus on holistic development and long-term capacity building—an approach that has been adopted in all AIDS-related planning during this period.

Empowering Civil Society Organisations

Civil society organisations play important roles in advocacy, participating in policy and programming design and implementation, and in the provision of services, especially at the community level. For example, a great deal of Brazil's success in HIV prevention is due to the country's 600-plus non-governmental and community organisations. For the past decade or more, these organisations have established needle-exchange schemes, distributed condoms, managed support groups and provided counselling. They have also kept HIV/AIDS in the public spotlight, providing essential political pressure when needed. In 1999, when the Health Ministry faced cuts to its budget for AIDS, tuberculosis and other diseases, these groups mobilised. Their street protests and other activities were widely covered in the press, and received strong support from some parliamentarians. In the end, the funding was restored.

A strong civil society flourishes in an environment in which the State allows for such non-governmental organisation participation. In an activist mode, civil society organisations must be empowered by law and daily practice to organise, publish and collect information, while having legal recourse to the courts and, if necessary, the option to demonstrate. As active participants in policy and programming design and implementation, they must be at the table, right from the beginning.

The recent development of the United Republic of Tanzania's national AIDS policy, for example, was based on widespread consultation with all ministries and a range of civil society organisations. One issue that benefited from the participation of civil society was the response in the workplace to HIV/AIDS. Representatives of the Ministry of Labour, and employers' and workers' organisations worked together to create policies based on the ILO Code of Practice. Important recent financial initiatives have also incorporated the role of civil society into design and implementation.

The World Bank's Multi-Country AIDS Programme for Africa explicitly aims to use non-governmental organisations as implementing partners for approximately 50 per cent of the funding provided. The recently-established Global Fund to Fight AIDS, Tuberculosis and Malaria requires country proposals to pass through Country Coordination Mechanisms', which should involve civil society.

The principle of the Greater Involvement of People Living with HIV/AIDS (GIPA) remains a cornerstone of multisectoral responses. Historically, in countries such as Australia, Brazil, Côte d'Ivoire, France, Norway, Thailand, Uganda and the United Kingdom, organisations of persons living with HIV/AIDS have helped draft national plans and tailor them for grassroots conditions. This is occurring in more and more countries, with heartening results. In Cambodia, for example, the establishment of a national network of persons living with HIV/AIDS in 2001 reflects a positive social environment that is very different from that of even two years ago.

The legitimacy of the network was confirmed by the government's recent decision to include representatives of persons living with HIV/AIDS in Cambodia's Country Coordination Mechanism. On a policy level, this is reflected in the new national strategic framework for a comprehensive and multisectoral response to HIV/ AIDS, 2001–2005', which explicitly endorses GIPA as an overriding principle of the national response.

Institutional Structures

Diverse institutional structures and arrangements need to be in place to turn political commitment and multisectoral participation into effective programming. National Strategic Plans are the main tools for prioritising and budgeting a country's HIV/AIDS activities, since they provide the operational framework for investing new and existing financial resources. They also serve as a map for implementing structures, and highlight where human and institutional capacity must be strengthened.

Planning and Implementation

In January 2001, UNAIDS carried out an assessment of country readiness in order to determine how to apply increased levels of funding to HIV/AIDS programmes. The 114 countries assessed were drawn from all regions. 'Readiness' was assessed according to the status of five core components: a national strategic AIDS plan; the capacity to operationalise the plan; detailed costing of the strategic plan; a monitoring and evaluation strategy; and mechanisms that can achieve coordination among governments, non-governmental organisations, the United Nations system and bilateral donors.

The results of the assessment found that the relatively high number of national strategic plans and coordination mechanisms reflects the progress that has been made in terms of political leadership and the commitment of governments to mobilise a response to AIDS. Approximately 100 countries were able to draft proposals for the Global Fund within about six weeks, largely thanks to the existence of strategic plans and coordination committees that could be easily adapted to the Global Fund's requirements.

In Africa, there remain only a handful of countries with no AIDS response. But, in many cases, plans are still in their early stages, and costing and monitoring elements are still being elaborated. In Asia, planning is generally well advanced; in the few exceptions, the lack of preparedness may reflect a relatively low priority assigned to AIDS activities because HIV prevalence is still low. European responses to HIV vary. In some cases, programmes are only now gearing up to deal with recent steep increases in HIV incidence. AIDS responses in the Americas are, in many cases, long-standing and comprehensive, although there are a few countries that still lag behind. Overall, fewer countries had costed plans, and fewer still had monitoring and evaluation systems set up to help manage and adjust the implementation of activities. These findings highlight the need to focus on capacity building for the management of programmes around the world.

While the review looked at preparedness, the results should not imply that resources must only go to the best-prepared countries: in some cases, the need is greatest precisely because the countries are ill-prepared to meet the challenges of AIDS.

National coordination

A national response based on strategic planning and multisectoral approaches is not a magic solution to all possible challenges. In fact, it could even trigger some new complications such as 'turf ' conflicts, unclear divisions of responsibility, competition over budget allocations, and inconsistencies between ministries and sectors. It is therefore essential to have in place solid national structures that coordinate high-level decisionmaking with the operational arms.

Over the past two years, several countries have made substantial progress in creating institutional arrangements to better coordinate and manage their national responses. Each has gone about this differently.

Côte d'Ivoire has created a HIV/AIDS Ministry, while Cambodia has a National Authority, which is an inter-ministerial body comprising of 15 ministries, the Cambodian Red Cross and provincial governments. Brazil's National Coordination Unit (located within the Ministry of Health) has been the model for some countries, while others have followed the approach established in the early 1990s by Thailand, appointing councils or commissions in the office of the president or prime minister.

In a number of African countries, presidents, prime ministers, or their deputies chair national councils. Some central Asian countries have adopted the same model. Kazakhstan, for example, has both Central and Regional Cross-sectoral Committees, chaired by the Deputy Prime Minister and Deputy Governors respectively. Whatever type of body is created, it requires technical expertise and sustained resources, and it should be set up with clear mandates, lines of accountability and appropriate staff.

Another useful coordinating mechanism is the United Nations Theme Group on HIV/AIDS, which strives to improve coherence among stakeholders involved in government-led responses. Theme Groups are the primary channel and vehicle for the United Nations system's collective support to, and collaboration with, countries. Since being set up in a few countries in 1996, many Theme Groups have evolved from forums for information-sharing into vehicles for mobilising political commitment, or for facilitating partnerships between national and international partners. In Central Asia and Eastern Europe, for example, 26 Theme Groups have been created, including those in Kosovo, Montenegro and Serbia. They have proved particularly useful in building bridges for multi-partner initiatives such as the region's Inter-Agency Group on Young People's Health, Development and Protection.

Similarly, the coordinating councils of non-governmental organisations have helped avoid duplication, prioritise action, and add greater weight to advocacy work. Uruguay now has a National AIDS Non-governmental Organisations Forum that can provide greater coherence to Non-governmental organisation activities around the country. The Forum will maintain close ties with the Ministry of Health's National Coordination Unit. Similar structures are being formed in Argentina and Paraguay.

Decentralisation and Local Responses

In addition to developing coordination mechanisms, countries need efficient mechanisms for decentralising services. This is to ensure that national responses are effective throughout each country, in both urban and rural areas. District-level responses have emerged as prominent decentralisation tools. In countries where the district is the administrative unit closest to individual communities, it can serve as a bridge between community efforts and national strategic planning, and as a site for multisectoral planning.

Capacity Development

Developing the capacity to implement and manage the necessary programmes is crucial. In some places, a generalised lack of capacity hampers development activities, particularly in societies emerging from conflict or profound political change.

Almost everywhere, though, some capacity exists in most areas of prevention, treatment, care and impact mitigation. And that capacity can be enhanced. The greatest needs are in sub-Saharan Africa.

A variety of initiatives exist to meet these needs, including programmes by UNDP and the World Bank to improve public administration on a wide scale, and the efforts of WHO to improve health systems' performance. Other initiatives deal directly with capacity to manage AIDS programming, such as the Regional AIDS Training Network of Eastern and Southern Africa. The Network links 17 training institutions across the region to provide a range of courses for middle-level managers, supervisors and trainers from public institutions, non-governmental organisations, and the private sector. It also provides training for teachers, religious leaders and officials in government ministries, along with managers of factories, commercial firms and decision-makers in the private sector.

Training and skill-building are key components of capacity development. But boosting the human capacity needed to get the job done requires people with the necessary skills and expertise, along with environments conducive to maintaining and building capacity. The UNAIDS Secretariat, in partnership with the US Agency for International Development, the World Bank Institute and others, has embarked on a bid to strengthen human capacity in countries worldwide. The aim is to gather technical guidance on how to take 'training' to further levels, and enable individuals and organisations to recruit, develop and keep skilled leadership for HIV/AIDS-related action.

In Eastern Europe and Central Asia, many countries inherited an extensive social and health infrastructure. But that capacity is not always equal to some of the special challenges thrown up by the epidemic, such as HIV prevention among vulnerable groups. To a large extent, national programmes are not yet able to fully monitor HIV among these groups, and they lack the personnel with the skills to implement effective interventions. Considerable government investment will be required for relevant training. Small-scale projects can build the evidence required for advocacy with governments and provide a basis for expanding activities aimed at preventing HIV infection among injecting drug users.

HIV SURVEILLANCE SYSTEMS

As the HIV/AIDS pandemic is composed of multiple and dynamic epidemics, national as well as international agencies are adopting and modifying HIV surveillance systems to meet the specific needs of each epidemic. Methods and surveillance activities in a country with a predominantly heterosexual epidemic differ greatly from surveillance activities in a country where HIV infection is mostly found among men who have sex with men or injecting drug users.

UNAIDS, in collaboration with National AIDS Programmes, WHO, and other partners conducted a second generation surveillance project—'Surveillance on HIV/AIDS'—in eight countries in Africa, Asia and Latin America between 1999 and 2002. The project, executed by UNAIDS, is being implemented by the National AIDS Programmes and partners at country level, and aims to implement second generation HIV surveillance in eight countries in Africa, Asia and Latin America. The guidelines and recommendations given in this chapter are based on the experience gained from the project.

The principles of second generation surveillance aim to improve the quality of the information tracked by National AIDS Programmes. The main objective of second generation surveillance is to monitor HIV and high-risk behaviour trends over time in order to provide essential data needed for the development of interventions and the evaluation of their impact. Therefore, there needs to be effective coordination between the surveillance and prevention programmes.

The main recommendations for second generation surveillance can be summarised as follows:

i) In generalised epidemics where HIV prevalence is over 1 per cent of the general population, surveillance systems should concentrate on monitoring HIV infection and high-risk behaviour in the general population, and also include groups such as sex workers.

ii) In concentrated epidemics where HIV is over 5 per cent in any subpopulation at higher risk of infection (such as drug injectors, sex workers, men who have sex with men), surveillance systems should monitor infection and behaviour in those groups, paying particular attention to behavioural links between members of those groups and the general population. Groups linking subpopulations at higher risk of infection with the general population are called 'bridging populations'.

iii) In low-level epidemics where relatively low HIV prevalence (less than 5 per cent in any subpopulation) is measured in any group, surveillance systems focus largely on behaviours and HIV infection in groups at high risk, looking for changes in behaviour that may lead to an increase in the rate of infection.

Second generation surveillance is built upon a country's existing data collection system. Therefore, there is a need to evaluate the surveillance system, identifying what worked and which gaps remain. Once the limitations of the current system are identified, it becomes easier to elaborate a national plan for surveillance. National plans involve several key partners and professionals in order to implement these plans. An important step, therefore, and one of the best approaches to reaching a consensus for a sound surveillance plan, is to discuss the country's needs with the main partners involved in surveillance so that agreement can be reached about how to improve the information system.

Second generation surveillance aims to improve the quality and diversity of information sources. In order to achieve that, standard and rigorous study protocols have to be developed and implemented using appropriate methods and tools. The monitoring and evaluation of surveillance activities facilitate this process.

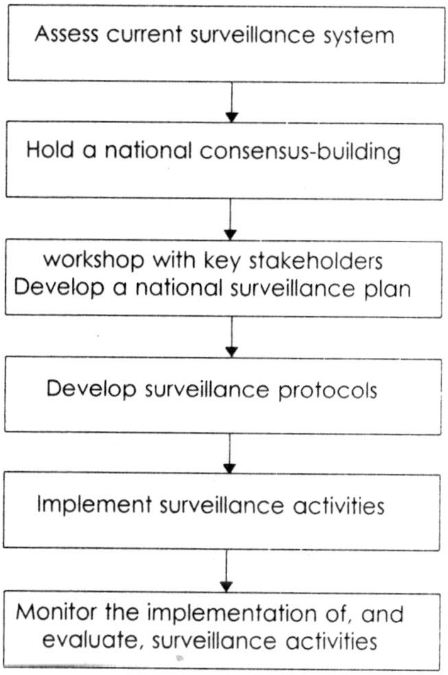

Figure 1. Framework for implementing HIV second generation surveillance: practical steps

Since 1999, UNAIDS, WHO and other international organisations have proposed a set of principles to improve a country's response to its HIV/AIDS epidemic. The framework for achieving this has been a shift from a health-sector approach to a multisectoral approach. Many countries are in the process of establishing, or have established, National Strategic Plans to expand their response to the epidemic. Strategic planning defines the general strategies, the institutional framework and the steps and activities needed to mobilise society as a whole to prevent and mitigate HIV infection. Strategic planning is a flexible tool designed to respond to changing situations, their objectives and, therefore, the activities to be implemented. It uses a decentralisation process as a way of ensuring that the needs at the community and local levels are met. There are three basic steps in establishing a national strategic plan:

i) situation and response analyses;
ii) plan formulation; and
iii) resource mobilisation.

To conduct a situation analysis, it is important to know who is infected with HIV, and who is vulnerable to infection, as well as identifying the main determinants of the HIV epidemic. This information is collected through second generation surveillance systems. In contrast to a traditional analysis, a situation analysis looks further into the social, economic and cultural contexts of HIV transmission. Ultimately, this will help clarify priorities and scopes of intervention. Even though there are underlying factors that lead people to engage in risky behaviour that can expose them to HIV, the epidemiological factors are the final determinants in explaining how HIV is spread. For example, are sex workers (SWs) also intravenous drug users (IDUs)? What are their behaviours and relationships with their clients, friends or partner(s)? The answers to these questions will lead to the planning of prevention programmes and contribute to the monitoring of their success.

The general objective of the national strategic planning process is that of contributing to countries' efforts to adapt to changing situations and to plan for, and effectively implement, efficient, affordable, sustainable, equitable and relevant expanded responses. To measure the progress and impact of these objectives, a monitoring and evaluation (M&E) system should be developed and put in place. An M&E system tracks what is being done and whether programmes are making a difference. It allows programme managers to calculate how to allocate resources in order to achieve the best overall result.

UNAIDS, WHO, UNICEF and their main partners have developed a Guide to Monitoring and Evaluation for National AIDS Programmes, in which the main indicators are selected according to the state of a country's epidemic. The list of indicators is not exhaustive but several core and additional indicators are listed with regard to monitoring progress and achievements. They are given below.

- Policy
- Condom availability and quality
- Stigma and discrimination
- Knowledge
- Voluntary counselling and testing
- Mother-to-child transmission
- Sexual negotiation and attitudes
- Sexual behaviour (includes that of men who have sex with men and that of sex workers)
- Young people's sexual behaviour
- Injecting drug use
- Blood safety/nosocomial transmission
- STI prevention and care
- Care and support
- Health and social impact

Second generation HIV surveillance systems will provide basic information for some of the programme areas of the National Strategic Plans. It is not an isolated system, but an important component that contributes to the understanding of the dynamics of HIV in the country context. These systems provide basic information for focusing and designing interventions as well as for monitoring the impact of interventions proposed within the strategic planning process. Information from these systems will provide decision-makers with key elements that will help them understand the impact of the prevention activities in different populations.

Assessment

Most countries have established national HIV/AIDS surveillance systems with varying degrees of success. Sexually transmitted infections (STIs) are regularly reported either as syndromes or etiologies by the standard health information system. Demographic health surveys (DHS), knowledge, attitude, practice and behaviour (KABP) studies or other kinds of behavioural studies may have been conducted. Therefore, the first step is to identify what has been done in the past and what is currently being done regarding the monitoring of HIV infection and its sexual determinants.

The objective of assessing surveillance systems is to analyse the relevance of the information collected by the different subsystems, in relation to the epidemic's state, and the use of this information. The ultimate goal of the assessment is to identify the strengths, limitations, problems and gaps in the system in order to plan activities to improve the quality of information provided to the NAP and its relevant partners. It is very important that NAPs, donors and other key stakeholders that are involved in surveillance activities or sexual behaviour studies agree on the objectives in order to join forces on a common agenda instead of carrying out independent ad hoc studies.

Even the most simplified surveillance systems have many components that need to be coordinated in order to collect relevant information. Not all countries have conducted regular evaluations of their surveillance systems. In many countries, surveillance activities have been conducted routinely, repeating the same survey every year, rather than adapting the HIV surveillance system to meet the needs created by the evolving epidemic. In order to build a better surveillance system, the most relevant strengths and weaknesses of the system must be identified so that any gaps can be filled in.

Sometimes an assessment is confused with an evaluation. Although they have similar objectives, they are slightly different. Assessments are usually a faster process, allowing for rapid action, and they require less input and information than do evaluations. Assessments attempt to collect basic information about the most relevant issues, whereas evaluations review all the elements in much more detail, require larger teams, use more in-depth analysis of the system, and therefore require more resources and time to obtain and release the information.

The main components of an assessment are summarised in below.

- Review documents (including protocols).
- Discuss with experts group (e.g. in-country national and international experts in surveillance).
- Interview key informants.
- Visit sites that conduct surveillance activities.
- Summarise and discuss main findings with NAP and partners.
- Share findings with key partners.

Some NAPs have conducted regular or periodic evaluations of the HIV surveillance systems, using the information obtained as an important basis for the development of second generation surveillance systems in the country. In countries where such evaluations have not taken place for three or four years, a rapid assessment of the HIV/AIDS/STI and behavioural studies surveillance system is necessary. Rapid assessments should be repeated every two-to-three years so as to regularly adjust the system in accordance with the changing epidemic.

Assessment of Sentinel Serosurveillance Systems

The rapid assessment of sentinel serosurveillance systems (HIV and STI) is carried out in four or five days by a small team of three-to-five people, maximum, and uses simple instruments. The outcome is a brief 10-20-page report, usually available within one month of the review. This contrasts with other reviews, which are more costly and complex and the results of which are often only available six months or more after the review has been carried out. There are different ways to conduct an assessment. For example, it can be done through a survey. A questionnaire is prepared with the most relevant questions regarding the surveillance system. This questionnaire is addressed to the persons involved in the surveillance system at the different levels and bilateral and multilateral cooperation agencies involved in surveillance activities. Information is then collected and analysed.

Different questionnaires need to be developed because of the differing partners and levels of involvement in the surveillance system. For example, the questions for national epidemiologists will differ from the questions for the laboratory personnel or health personnel collecting the blood samples. Another approach, equally effective and more expedient, is to review documents related to surveillance activities, such as surveillance protocols and reports, and to conduct interviews of the key personnel involved in implementing the HIV surveillance system.

Small group discussions are carried out with NAP personnel and key informants from the main partners involved in surveillance. This method provides enough information for the assessment team to have a clear understanding of what the level of performance is and the efficiency of the HIV surveillance system. At the same time, it will help to identify the main partners or possible partners involved in surveillance activities. This information helps later on in the process of building up a consensus for an improved surveillance system.

An important aspect of the assessment is to verify whether surveillance activities are carried out according to the procedures described in the surveillance protocol. During visits to the sentinel surveillance sites and laboratories, the conditions in which samples are collected and analysed can be observed. As an example, in one country, the surveillance guidelines established that anonymous, unlinked tests were collected for surveillance among pregnant women. When one of the sentinel sites was visited, however, it was found that the health centre had a log book with the names of the women whose blood had been collected and the HIV results provided by the laboratory, obviously breaking the anonymity provided by unlinked, anonymous testing. A lack of supervision by the person responsible at the central level was one reason why this occurred.

Whether a more formal evaluation process, a situation analysis that is done as part of the national strategic plan, or a rapid assessment is used, the main components of the second generation surveillance system need to be reviewed. The components to be reviewed in the assessment process include:

- HIV/AIDS/STI surveillance framework
- AIDS/HIV infection case reporting
- Sentinel surveillance for HIV
- Surveillance for STI
- Laboratory practices and quality assessment
- Behavioural studies
- Other relevant HIV/AIDS studies or sources of information in the country
- Management of the system, including information
- Resources
- Analysis, dissemination and use of information

The assessment does not need to look at these components in a sequential fashion, but it must be effective in examining all the components and addressing all the issues relevant to surveillance. It is essential that the national context and the development activities of the National AIDS Programme be understood, and that responsibilities for specific surveillance activities be clearly identified.

One possible way to review, present and summarise the assessment results is through an analysis that focuses on the strengths, weaknesses, opportunities and threats (SWOT). The SWOT analysis provides a good framework for identifying the strengths and limitations of the surveillance system.

In order to improve the quality of information and performance of the system, the opportunities identified in the country will need to overcome any constraints on the system. Gaps and weaknesses in the system need to be identified so that they can be resolved. This type of analysis should be carried out for each component (HIV/AIDS, STI, sexual behaviour studies). The analysis of each component will be included in a final SWOT analysis to provide an overall picture.

Other rapid assessment methodologies can be used as well. But the basic principle is that the appropriate methods and tools are kept simple in order to achieve quick results and collect the key information. Another way to present the results is to name and enumerate the limitations and constraints of the surveillance system according to the different levels of the system, its functions and responsibilities. Although sometimes the roles and responsibilities are not well defined for each level, the assessment team needs to obtain a clear idea of what these are.

The rapid assessment process encourages a participatory approach at these different levels and the findings are immediately discussed in small groups or meetings in which self-critiquing is encouraged in order to initiate changes. Using either the SWOT analysis or other approaches, the results should provide summarised information to National AIDS Programme managers or donors who may then use them to make decisions regarding surveillance activities and any gaps or limitations that need to be overcome.

Assessment of Behavioural Surveillance System

Behavioural surveillance is a core component of second generation surveillance. This review can be undertaken in addition to the previous rapid assessment described, or can take place concurrently. It is useful when assessing the surveillance system to review all behavioural surveillance that has been carried out and the number of studies conducted in the country in the past four or five years. The review aims to:

1) draw up an inventory of studies carried out to date;
2) understand behavioural trends among the general population and vulnerable groups, based on the behavioural indicators used and populations studied;
3) identify gaps both in the data on these populations and in the indicators used;
4) identify the pool of expertise (institutions and individuals in the country).

The following information needs to be collected in order to review the state of the art of behavioural studies:

— Author's name
— Title
— Date
— Type of study and location
— Group(s) studied and ages
— Sample size
— Indicators used and main findings
— Strengths
— Limitations

This behavioural review can be done by an in-country consultant as a data-collection exercise. It should take one-to-two weeks. One week should be sufficient to analyse the data and to obtain basic information on behavioural studies. Suggested categories for the analyses are: vulnerable groups; title, authors, date, reference; institution(s) in charge of study design, data collection, analysis; methodology and main findings by determinants/factors.

Whatever tools or approaches are used to assess the HIV surveillance system, the main objective of the process is to identify what does and does not work in the system. Identifying strengths, weaknesses, opportunities and threats is one way to facilitate the planning process. The findings of the review of the HIV, STI and behavioural surveillance systems are specific to each country. It is useful for the programme managers and partners to understand and consolidate the positive aspects of their country's surveillance system and, in parallel, to identify the main gaps that need to be addressed. These steps, in turn, allow those involved to build on existing strengths, and to map out the opportunities for moving into a second generation HIV surveillance system.

Consensus-building

Today, epidemiology and information systems have gained increasing importance and are serve as the main driving forces behind programmes. Results of epidemiological studies are used to inform health professionals, the public and policy-makers about the need for new or different health policies. This process is the translation of epidemiological research into public health action. But sometimes translation does not take place, due to a variety of factors, such as poor communication, the lack of advocacy efforts by epidemiologists or a manager's lack of information. Second generation surveillance information systems should drive policies and translate information into action.

Following the review and assessment of the HIV surveillance systems, the NAP and all key stakeholders, including bilateral donors, NGOs and research institutions, need to agree on gaps and shortcomings and on methods for improving the surveillance system. They must also set priorities and identify who contributes to what, and when. This phase lays the foundation for the National Second Generation Surveillance Plan and facilitates the coordination process with all the partners involved in surveillance activities.

Consequently, the different partners can identify how they can contribute financially or technically to the systems, thereby increasing the system's sustainability.

All key partners involved in surveillance are invited to a national consensus-building workshop aimed at developing a common vision of how to improve surveillance in the country. The outcome of this workshop will vary according to the particular situation in each country. For example, a country may need only to review its protocol and update it with new recommendations. But other countries may need to outline a national surveillance plan to raise resources or shift HIV surveillance to other groups.

Ideally, workshop participants aim to develop the draft of a national surveillance plan that encompasses HIV, STI and behavioural components. Countries may also choose to draft a broader monitoring and evaluation plan that encompasses various essential HIV-related programmes, in addition to all the surveillance components.

The major programme areas for monitoring and evaluation include:

i) HIV/STI and syphilis surveillance
ii) Monitoring of sexual behaviour
iii) STI care and prevention
iv) Voluntary counselling and testing services
v) Blood safety
vi) Monitoring of condom availability and accessibility

The consensus-building workshop for second generation surveillance aims to reach broad agreement among the main partners on the key issues and information needed with regard to HIV surveillance. It is important to have a clear idea of the outcome expected from such an exercise. For that, it is essential that the objectives and process required for achieving such results be clearly outlined in the planning document. The expected outcomes of a national consensus building workshop can be summarised as follows:

— identify the M&E indicators and surveillance strategy to measure the objectives of the National Strategic Plan;
— identify the main populations, methods and indicators to be used in second generation surveillance;
— consolidate a draft outline of an action plan for implementing second generation surveillance, including that of HIV, AIDS, STI and behaviour among different populations; and
— review the surveillance tools.

The participants in the consensus-building process should be the individuals, organisations and institutions that are involved in HIV surveillance activities. Participants may vary in different situations, but the main groups involved are: government, multilateral and bilateral organisations, NGOs, universities and research institutions, and epidemiologists and social scientists who are usually directly involved in collecting information. Relevant donors and stakeholders should also participate to determine the information needs. To ensure success, the objectives should be agreed upon by all participants.

The implementation experience in different countries has shown that the consensus-building workshop agenda varies considerably from one country to another, based on the various countries' status and priorities. The agenda therefore needs to be tailored to each country, and may even be modified during the workshop. The workshop comprise working groups in which participants discuss the best strategy for improving the system. Consensus is then reached in plenary sessions with national and international partners on how to move ahead on second generation surveillance.

The essential steps for reaching consensus become increasingly complex as the workshop progresses. At a minimum, during the consensus-building workshop, the participants need to agree on the following aspects:

i) review the principles and rationale for the second generation surveillance, and for subsystems;
ii) review the findings and recommendations from the assessment and reach a common vision of the second generation surveillance system;
iii) describe the experiences and limitations of the present surveillance system;
iv) identify the populations to be surveyed;
v) identify the sites or locations for each type of population;
vi) select the indicators to be used for each population;
vii) present the existing multisectoral national HIV/ AIDS/STI plans, or equivalent;
viii) if an M&E plan is developed, select indicators for the main activities for each component of the M&E plan including a national HIV plan;
ix) identify the methods and/or sources to be used to collect the indicators for each surveillance subsystem;
x) identify the partners to be involved from the different sectors;
xi) discuss draft protocols of surveillance (if they exist);
xii) agree on an implementation timetable and follow-up activities by partners, including financial contributions needed, with an estimated budget for two-to-three years; and
xiii) agree on monitoring and evaluations of surveillance.

Developing a National Surveillance Plan

Having a national surveillance plan is beneficial for several reasons. Over time, the plan will allow all stakeholders to develop a comprehensive and thorough understanding of the strategy of the NAP or the Ministry of Health. This will allow stakeholders to identify how they can best contribute-technically and financially to these efforts, and to complement each other, instead of duplicating efforts. The national surveillance plan also helps to legitimise surveillance as a worthwhile programme among many competing programmes, and allows for the findings to be entered into the National Strategic Plan.

Drafting of the national surveillance plan is the responsibility of the NAP, and should take place shortly after the consensus-building workshop. This would be followed by specific activities related to the implementation of the surveillance, i.e., protocol development. Surveillance indicators are part of the broader country monitoring-and-evaluation plans and, if integrated into an M&E plan, are better accepted, sustained and used by the NAP.

The key to successfully establishing a good surveillance system is consistency and systematisation of the process to develop the plan. Surveillance systems, both for HIV prevalence rates and behaviours, monitor trends in a cost-effective way. Therefore, the systems should monitor the same populations over time, in similar geographical locations, using the same tools to collect the information. This method contrasts with large population-based sample studies, which cannot be repeated too often because of their high costs.

The main elements of a national surveillance planned to contain at least the following component.

- Identification of the structure of surveillance unit, coordination, resource mobilisation and dissemination
- Priority areas of the National Strategic Plan, including the link between surveillance plan and strategic plan
- General strategy for HIV surveillance
- Main objectives
- Expected results
- Activities
- Identification of populations, locations and timeframes

— Surveillance among programme areas: HIV and syphilis, sexual behaviour, STI information
— Schedule of activities
— Resources needed
— Monitoring and evaluation of the surveillance system

At the same time, the system should be flexible enough if the results obtained are not relevant or do not provide good information. For example, in the case of a Latin American country, HIV surveillance had been carried out among pregnant women for the previous eight years. The surveillance systems showed a prevalence rate of less than 0.4 per cent among antenatal attendees. On the other hand, reported AIDS cases in the country showed that more than 60 per cent of cases were related to men who have sex with men (MSM), indicating that the surveillance system needs to strengthen reporting among this group.

Surveillance Protocols

Preparing specific surveillance protocols that contain the main elements of the system is an important step in the implementation of second generation HIV surveillance systems. Protocols ensure that the surveillance system is consistent over time, regardless of changes in personnel. These documents help to clarify the aims of the system and how it is integrated into the National Strategic Plan. Protocols are key elements in the coordination of surveillance activities among the various players. They serve as a history of the surveillance system's evolution for future use. And, finally, they serve as a quality-assurance mechanism; taking into account the high turnover of some NAP personnel, sound protocols guarantee consistency in the survey procedures. There should be specific protocols for each component of the system—HIV prevalence, sexual behaviour, HIV/AIDS cases and STIs.

A good protocol will ensure standard procedures for the collection of information, either on behaviour or HIV infection, across different sites and populations. Surveillance protocols should contain clear objectives regarding the information sought and should have well-defined indicators. This will allow for comparisons over time of some populations followed in similar locations.

It is advisable to have separate protocols for each component of the system: HIV seroprevalence among antenatal clinic attendees; HIV/AIDS cases; STIs; and sexual behaviour among the populations around the sentinel sites or among other at-risk populations. Whether a specific country has a low-level, concentrated or generalised epidemic, a surveillance protocol for each activity should include the following basic common components in order to be systematic and consistent:

i) *Definition of objectives.* What are the primary and specific objectives of the surveillance activity? Is the activity integrated into the more general context of the NAP and, if so, how? Is it integrated into the M&E plan and the National Strategic Plan?
ii) *Definition of indicators.* What are the essential indicators that have been identified and will be monitored over time?
iii) *Development and validation of tools and instruments. What* tools and instruments are needed for collecting information? Have the tools and instruments already been validated, or will they be? Do they have internal and external validation for the country? Have they been adapted to suit the local culture?
iv) *Implementation procedures.* How is the information going to be collected? Who is going to be responsible for collecting the information? Who does what, where and when?
v) *Data analysis and interpretation.* Who is responsible for analysing the data and interpreting the results?
vi) *Development of mechanisms to disseminate information.* Who is going to disseminate the information and how will this be done at local and national levels? When will it be done, and what are the target audiences?

vii) *Budget.* Who will pay for what?

viii) *Timeline.* When specific steps will be carried out?

The main components of a standard protocol for HIV surveillance are the following.

i) Justification

ii) Objectives

iii) Population, geographical area

iv) Description of methods:

  a) sampling methods

  b) information sources

  c) ethical aspects

  d) laboratory procedures

  e) collection of socio-demographic data

  f) quality control

v) Monitoring and supervision

vi) Data management and analysis

vii) Dissemination and use.

Protocols may need to be changed or revised over time in accordance with the results of the evaluation of the second generation surveillance systems. Other second generation guideline modules have been, or are being, developed, dealing in greater detail with such issues as the selection of populations, sampling methods, laboratory procedures, analysis and use of data.

Monitoring

Monitoring is the continuous management assessment of surveillance system implementation in relation to agreed protocol. It contributes to effective reporting and it focuses on the somewhat delicate process of supervision of protocol implementation or data collection. The most important part of monitoring is assessing whether the elements of the surveillance system are performing according to plan.

Monitoring is a continuous process and it should be conducted at all levels of the system. If there are clear and precise protocols for HIV surveillance, monitoring the HIV information system is relatively simple. HIV surveillance protocols should clearly outline the steps required for collecting information on HIV, STIs or behaviours.

Stakeholders are involved in the various stages of the country-driven process to develop and implement HIV/AIDS activities. Experience shows that it is worth taking the time to go through the process of achieving consensus fully and systematically rather than omitting some steps. For example, in some countries, implementation of surveys may occur more than a year after the initial assessment of the surveillance system. Nevertheless, ownership is achieved.

The implementation of surveillance activities is greatly facilitated by the common vision established by national and local programme managers, and partners involved in surveillance. There is a common feeling and understanding of what needs to be accomplished and how. The consensus-building workshops and transparency of the whole process will encourage the involvement of national institutions and strengthening of their capacities—for example, regional or national centres working on HIV issues, such as those in Thailand, have been involved in training for data collection of behavioural data. Countries have become conscious of the importance of encompassing behavioural surveillance within their systems, and have taken the necessary steps to implement these protocols.

A good surveillance study protocol is a necessary element for building a good information system but it is not enough in itself. If a good protocol is not well implemented, the information produced may be of poor quality. The sound implementation of protocols is essential in order to produce good information. For surveillance activities implementation this, it is necessary to have good instruments and, above all, a very good supervisory system.

In order to minimise potential biases, avoid mistakes in interpretation, human error, logistical constraints or any other unforeseen problem, there is a need to closely monitor the process of data collection. The best way to ensure that the protocol is respected and the information collected as planned is through supervision of the whole process.

Another advantage of monitoring the implementation of protocols is that it ensures the credibility of the information collected. Sometimes the information provided by a surveillance system may be questioned by some donors and authorities—even health ministers. If the quality of the system is ensured by close supervision, potential problems and misunderstandings can be avoided or confronted.

It is important that a full-time surveillance team be assigned to oversee the implementation and coordination of surveillance protocols, given the numerous partners and components involved in surveillance activities. The collection sites must be visited to ensure that information is collected adequately. For this, the supervisors need to be very familiar with the surveillance protocol and need to know the exact steps to be taken when collecting the information.

Monitoring focuses more on process indicators to show that activities are carried out in accordance with the protocol. But it also identifies problems so that immediate corrective action can be taken. The key point is that the final indicators produced by the information system are more robust if the system has performed as planned than if the quality was poor.

Instruments for collecting this information should be developed. Monitoring, as a continuous process, refers to the regular collection, analysis and use of information. It focuses more on the inputs, performance and progress of the information system. For example, a checklist for a supervisory visit can be prepared. This checklist should include general information about the sites, the number of samples collected versus the number expected, materials required, the supply of materials, etc. In brief, the checklist should include all the main elements of the established protocol.

Information is valuable in HIV planning and the monitoring of responses as long as it is of a high standard. One of the main tasks of national surveillance teams is to ensure that activities for surveillance are implemented according to the various protocols established to monitor the different determinants.

The ongoing process of monitoring the system during protocol implementation is vital to ensuring the overall accuracy of the study results. The study protocols should establish the various responsibilities for monitoring and supervision at the different levels. The quality of the results is therefore the responsibility of all levels of staff involved with the implementation of surveillance activities. The national coordinator or the national committee (the main parties responsible for surveillance activities) is primarily responsible for monitoring the compliance of methods outlined in the study protocols. Second generation surveillance promotes greater geographical and population coverage.

Regional or provincial and onsite coordinators should identify the gaps, constraints and problems in implementing the surveillance protocols and also play an active role in ensuring that the data are collected according to the defined protocols. For example, regular monitoring of the field operations should verify that the inclusion and exclusion criteria are fully respected. It should also ensure that sample sizes established for each population are completed in the stipulated time and that the principles of confidentiality and sound ethics are respected. Measures should also be taken to monitor the accuracy of data being collected and entered into the data management system. If blood samples are taken, the recently published guidelines for using HIV testing technologies in surveillance can be consulted for more detailed and useful information on how to proceed with HIV testing.

For data management, it is important that appropriate training be carried out for those responsible for completing the forms or questionnaires and entering the data on computer. Feedback to all staff involved in the implementation of HIV surveillance activities at the different levels is also essential and may be done through a publication or a one-day workshop. A multidisciplinary technical working/reference group for HIV/AIDS and STI surveillance has been found to be very useful in some countries, enhancing the overall acceptability and credibility of surveillance results at national and international level.

Evaluation

Evaluation involves the periodic assessment of the HIV surveillance system's performance efficiency. It reveals which components of the system are strong and which need to be strengthened in order to improve the quality of the information. Involving indepth analysis of the HIV information system, evaluation is aimed at determining whether the goals of the surveillance system have been met.

Evaluation is the careful examination of an ongoing or completed project. It is a one-step process and takes into account not only the design of the surveillance system but also its implementation and results. It should be planned from the beginning of the activity. An evaluation should address the following key issues:

i) Are the goals and objectives of the HIV surveillance system clearly stated?
ii) Are there standard protocols for the mechanisms used to collect information?
iii) How effective were the various components of the system (data collection, laboratory facilities, questionnaires used, etc.)?
iv) What are the human and financial resources used, and the direct and indirect costs involved?

v) Is the acquired information being used and adequately disseminated?

Sharing information is as important as collecting the data. If the data are not reliable or properly collected, the information provided by the surveillance system is of little use. A good HIV surveillance system should include the basic elements of M&E to reassure the partners and authorities that the data collected are meaningful, since different decisions will be made according to the quality of data. It is always advisable to provide arguments that build trust in the HIV surveillance system so that any decisions made are known to have been based on reliable information.

Evaluation of second generation surveillance systems should be tailored to the country and its specific HIV situation. Scientific rigour must be combined with practical realities. The frequency and scope of evaluation will depend on factors such as the level of satisfaction, performance of the system and resources available.

Evaluations are usually conducted on a periodic basis and can take one of the following forms:

i) an internal, annual, rapid evaluation, by national experts
ii) an external biannual or tri-annual evaluation, by external experts
iii) a combination of external and internal expert evaluation.

An intermediate step towards improving HIV surveillance systems could take the form of an evaluation workshop. The results of HIV surveillance systems are then disseminated and shared with the appropriate audiences, including, ideally, the participants and technical staff involved in the survey. During this dissemination workshop, a participatory assessment could be carried out in cooperation with the technical staff and main partners involved. The problems and limitations of the surveillance system are exposed and solutions proposed. In this workshop, results are presented and reviewed and recommendations made to improve the next round of surveys. This process of reviewing surveillance results, monitoring reports and obtaining feedback from participants at all levels enhances the quality of future surveillance surveys.

REFERENCES

Bloom, S.S., et al., "Looking for change in response to the AIDS epidemic: Trends in AIDS knowledge and sexual behaviour in Zambia, 1990 through 1998", *Journal of Acquired Immune Deficiency Syndromes*; 25(1): 77–85.

Cohen, D., *Mainstreaming the policy and programming response to the HIV epidemic*, New York, UNDP, 2000.

Coombe, C., *Managing the impact of HIV/AIDS on the education sector*, University of Pretoria: Centre for the study of AIDS, 2000.

Desmond C., Michael K, Gow J., *The Hidden Battle: HIV/AIDS in the Family and Community*, Health Economics and HIV/AIDS Research Division (HEARD). Durban: University of Natal, 2001.

FAO, *The impact of HIV/AIDS on food security*, 2001.

Fylkesnes, K., et al., "Declining HIV prevalence and risk behaviours in Zambia: evidence from surveillance and population-based surveys", *AIDS*; 15(7): 907–916, 2001.

Ghys P., et al., "HIV surveillance among female sex workers", *AIDS*; 15(3): 33–34, 2001.

Salama ,P., Dondero, T., "HIV surveillance in complex emergencies", *AIDS*; 15(3): S4–12.

UNAIDS, *United Nations-Facilitated Response to HIV/AIDS, STD and Drug Use in Central Asian Countries*, (Kazakhstan, Kyrgyzstan, Tajikistan, Turkmenistan and Uzbekistan), Geneva, 1999.

______________ *UN System Strategic Plan for HIV/AIDS – 2001 to 2005*, Geneva, 2000.

______________ *HIV/AIDS, Schools and Education Global Strategy Framework*, Geneva, 2001.

8

HIV/AIDS in India

HIV/AIDS has quickly emerged as one of the most serious public health problems in the country with infections currently being reported in all states and territories. India has the largest number of people living with HIV/AIDS in Asia. Globally, it is second only to South African in terms of the overall number of people living with the disease.

The first case of AIDS in India was detected in 1986. According to UNAIDS estimates of 2001, 3.97 million Indians were HIV positive. However, due to the country's large population, the high number of infections translates into a relatively low adult prevalence of 0.8 per cent. One per cent increase in prevalence could add 5 million new infections. Health officials concede that these estimates represent only a fraction of total AIDS morbidity in India. Some experts believe the number of individuals infected with HIV/AIDS in India is actually much higher.

Common opportunistic infections (OIs) associated with the reported cases of AIDS in India have been tuberculosis, fungal infection of the mouth (oral candidiasis), *Cryptosporidia* (causing diarrhoea), *Pnuemocystis carineii* (causing pneumonia) and *Herpes Zoster* (causing shingles). While a detailed account of the economic burden of treating different episodes of these OIs at the family level and in hospital settings are yet to be worked out, it has been documented that satellite epidemics of OIs are happening in different parts of the country. Managing the dual epidemic of tuberculosis and HIV/AIDS is currently posing a great challenge to the public health practitioners. HIV prevalence ranging from 10 to 20 per cent has been recorded among samples of urban TB patients in India, and it is projected that 20-25 per cent of the increase in TB cases over the next five years could be directly attributable to co-infection.

Table 1. Estimated number of people living with HIV/AIDS (2001)

Estimated number of adults and children living with HIV/AIDS (end 2001)	3,970,000
Total population (2001)	1,025,096,000
Adult HIV prevalence (end 2001)	0.8%
HIV-1 sero-prevalence in urban areas	
Population most at risk (i.e., sex workers and clients, patients seeking care for a sexually transmitted infection, or others with known risk factors)	4.8%
Population not at risk (i.e., pregnant women, blood donors, or others with no known risk factors)	0.1%

Sources: UNAIDS, U.S. Census Bureau

HIV INFECTION: TRENDS ACROSS STATES

No single state or union territory in India is free from HIV. The states and union territories can be broadly classified into three groups based on the different stages of development of the HIV epidemic. They are:

i) *States with generalised HIV epidemic*: In this category are included Maharashtra, Tamil Nadu, Karnataka, Andhra Pradesh, Manipur and Nagaland where HIV prevalence has reached 1 per cent in antenatal clinic attending women representing female general population. While the first outbreak of HIV infection happened among injection heroin users in the north-eastern states of Manipur and Nagaland which have common borders with Myanmar, the other states in this category had seen the epidemic taking off first among female sex workers. However, all the states subsequently saw a significant progress of HIV in general population. HIV care and management-needs are pressing issues now in these states on top of prevention, as increasing numbers of AIDS deaths, young widows and AIDS orphans on the one hand and increased hospital bed occupancy for HIV disease on the other, are being recorded.

ii) *Concentrated HIV epidemic states*: HIV has infected more than 5 per cent of the population groups observing high-risk behaviour in these states but the prevalence in female general population has remained below 1 per cent. Gujarat, Goa, Pondicherry, Mizoram and West Bengal fall in this category. The epidemic is making in-roads in bridge population such as migrant labourers and clients of female sex workers in these states. It is still not clear what are the best ways to intervene in these populations, essentially due to lack of evidence on best practices. It is important to note that although HIV epidemic took off at the same time in IDUs in three north-eastern states (Manipur, Mizoram and Nagaland), the subsequent course taken by the virus was different, as reflected by the current sentinel surveillance data. While Manipur and Nagaland have seen a rise in HIV in IDUs followed by a rise in HIV prevalence in antenatal clinic attending women, Mizoram saw a plateauing of HIV epidemic among IDUs around 5 per cent, and HIV prevalence among heterosexuals went up. It is important to identify the determinants of this heterogeneity in different north-eastern states for effective future interventions.

iii) *Low HIV epidemic*: Remaining states and union territories fall in this category where the population groups observing high-risk behaviour is yet to attain a 5 per cent prevalence of HIV. While these could be seen as states having windows of opportunity for preventing an intense HIV epidemic, one needs to also examine whether the required coverage is being met under the sentinel surveillance. For example, the National AIDS Control Organisation (NACO)

> sees strengthening of sentinel surveillance in Assam, Bihar and Orissa as an issue of urgent importance, since in many rounds of sentinel surveillance the requisite number of samples tested (denominator) could not be collected. Although Tripura – the smallest northeastern state of India – which has common border with Bangladesh, has reported low HIV and limited injection drug use, anecdotal data reveals an established route for cross border smuggling of injection tidigesic (buprenorphine) ampoules from India to Bangladesh. On the other hand, Meghalaya has reported mostly oral dextropropoxyphene, diazepam and nitrazepam use and limited heroin smoking and still lower injecting practices among local youths as well as students coming from other northeastern states to Shillong (the capital of Meghalaya) for pursuing higher studies. A regional approach to designing innovative interventions is therefore required where AusAID and Sida have taken some important initiatives. However, there are states in north-east India such as Arunachal Pradesh, Tripura and Assam that are yet to get adequate attention from donor agencies for designing of intervention low prevalence setting. Similarly, diffusion of injection drug use occurring in other metropolitan cities of India outside the northeast, require urgent attention too.

While the socio-economic impact is directly linked to the magnitude of the epidemic, the extent of devastation caused by it can be gleaned from a very early study done by Bloom and Glied. This study estimated that there will be a total of 1 million AIDS cases by the year 2000, yielding a total of $11 billion in direct and indirect costs. Direct costs include medical costs whereas indirect costs comprise value of income foregone because of AIDS-related morbidity and mortality.

The AIDS surveillance system in India is in a nascent stage compared to the HIV surveillance system, and thus the reported cumulative AIDS cases of 20,304 greatly understates the real number of AIDS cases in India, and therefore will also understate the macro costs of the epidemic. Evidence indicates that at least 40 per cent of the patients reporting for the first time in OPDs in apex hospitals, are in advanced stages of AIDS, and are being missed out at the district levels. Thus, the figure of 1 million AIDS cases in 2000 may be much closer to the actual load of AIDS cases in the country.

A more recent study is the one by Murray and Lopez of the Burden Of Disease in India, the World Bank, where they have calculated the trends in Disability Adjusted Life Years (DALYs) lost due to selected diseases in four States (Andhra Pradesh, Karnataka, Punjab and West Bengal) of India. The study indicates that communicable diseases still predominate in terms of disease burden, especially in the young age groups. A projection till 2020 based on alternative assumptions indicate that DALYs lost due to HIV infections in India are expected to rise significantly up to the year 2010 and decline thereafter.

The impact of the epidemic is likely to be felt on all sectors: households, communities, industry, agriculture, health as well as the government. A study that looked at the economic impact on individuals who were HIV positive indicated that the group on an average spent between 10 to 30 per cent of their annual incomes on HIV-related health expenditures, with the bulk of expenditures being on drugs and medicines. As expected, individuals with lower income as well as with at least one child had a greater probability of a more severe impact than others did. The immediate implication of this is that economic impact will be most severely felt by households that are relatively less well off and have a greater number of dependents.

The 1997 World Bank report on Confronting AIDS states that if India maintains its current level of health care subsidies, a severe AIDS epidemic would increase government expenditure by about $2 billion per year by 2010. If subsidies are increased to the 50 per cent level, the same size epidemic would increase annual government health expenditure by an additional $30 billion.

Another study which looked at the health and treatment costs for 1999 calculated that Rs. 2,045 crores would have been spent in 1999 in India, which translates into about $95 million in current prices. This was the minimum expenditures or costs that would have taken place in one year if only 2.8 per cent of the individuals are on antiretroviral treatment and only half of the new infections in 1999 display any opportunistic infection. Clearly, this kind of expenditure is untenable for a country like India, irrespective of who spends the money.

The socio-economic impact will be felt at both the individual and household level, but also at the macro and sectoral level. The two sectors that are most severely going to be affected are the health and the government sectors. The health sector will increasingly see a rise in demand for health care, and given the current health sector scenario, pressures on existing government hospitals will rise; there is already evidence of this from states like Tamil Nadu and Manipur. This is bound to have impact on individuals accessing health care for other diseases as AIDS care can crowd out not-AIDS care.

The government will also need to think strategically about its policy on newer treatments like anti retroviral therapy (ART), which are now seen as being central to the treatment of HIV positive patients. The issue around ART has become even more critical since the prices of these drugs have been falling, indicting a possibility of subsidizing these drugs. The fact that most of the major drug companies manufacturing these drugs are Indian has made this issue even more sensitive in India.

Given India's low per capita income, as well as competing needs outside health sector – and within the health sector – it is not clear to what extent the government can subsidize ART. At the same time, greater access to ART will clearly reduce health expenditures and reduce economic impact at all levels. by keeping individuals healthy and productive. This is an area. which has yet to see much policy-oriented analysis.

While most of the public health experts and social scientists in the country believe that HIV is not going to take a course similar to the one that happened in Africa, the epidemiological evidence obtained so far does ring an alarm of concern. The virus in India has taken different courses in different states since its first detection in 1986 in Chennai, and has contributed to the heterogeneous picture of the epidemic within the country. Of course, this heterogeneity has been influenced by varied sexual and injection behaviour patterns among network population groups as well as 'bridge population' linking different networks.

Genesis and extent of response to the epidemic differed across states, and played their role in shaping the epidemic differently in different states. It is important to note that the number of people living with HIV in South and South-East Asia is dominated by India; in 2001, 63 per cent of the Asia-Pacific total estimate of 6.1 million People Living with HIV (PLWH) were in this country alone.

The estimated number of people living with HIV in the country was 3.5 million, 3.7 million, 3.86 million and 3.97 million respectively in 1998, 1999, 2000 and 2001. These estimates have used HIV sentinel surveillance data collected from antenatal clinic attending women, STD clinic attendees, injecting drug users and men having sex with men. Altogether 237 select sites were used for this purpose from all over the country, of which 109 were STD clinics, 110 clinics for pregnant women, 11 sites for injecting drug users (IDUs) and only two for men having sex with men (MSM).

AIDS cases were not included at the time of calculating the estimates using sentinel surveillance data, and the age range in focus was 15 to 49 years. Also, sex workers are not currently being included as a sentinel group in the surveillance. Lack of adequate representation of all the risk groups as well as lack of proper geographic spread — including proper representation from rural areas — in sentinel surveillance, clearly highlight the need for involving these sub-populations and non-government organisations having active contact with some of the 'hard to reach population' such as IDUs and MSMs in surveillance activities.

WAYS OF HIV TRANSMISSION

In India, 75 to 80 per cent of HIV transmission is through heterosexual sex. HIV prevalence rates are highest among sex workers and their clients. The latter, in turn, take the disease back to their homes and infect their wives. Mobile populations, notably truckers, have been especially important in spreading the disease. Apart from sex workers and truckers, high-risk populations include migrant labourers, prisoners, and military troops stationed in remote areas, especially in the north-east.

Sex work

A countrywide surveillance for HIV was initiated in 1985 by the apex research institute ICMR. This generated the first evidence for presence of HIV from a group of female sex workers in Chennai in 1986. Subsequently HIV prevalence in sex workers in Mumbai went up from 0 per cent in 1987 to 20 per cent within a period of three years. All these early cross-sectional findings prompted launching of targeted interventions in brothel based sex workers in different parts of India, especially since evidence from successful AIDS control projects around the world showed targeted intervention approach to be able to stop the transmission of infection within and from the 'core transmitters'. However, adequate knowledge of the vulnerability of certain population groups such as unorganised sector of sex workers to HIV and STD is still lacking. Thus, it is not clear how exactly to reduce risks in these hard-to-reach populations, and what would comprise effective intervention for these groups.

Drug use

During the initial phase of HIV epidemic in India, injection drug use related HIV was identified from the north-eastern States of Manipur, Mizoram and Nagaland, which had a common international border with Myanmar; the drug of choice for injecting was heroin. The HIV prevalence in local IDUs in Manipur, Mizoram and Nagaland subsequently stabilised at 80 per cent, 5 per cent and 50 per cent respectively.

Although the present scenario of drug use in the country has changed considerably, the State AIDS Prevention and Control Societies in the states other than the North-East are yet to support outreach and harm reduction activities. Recent data from the 'Rapid Situation Assessment' reveal that a diffusion of injection drug use has taken place in major metropolitan cities of Kolkata, Delhi, Chennai and Mumbai, as well as in other parts of India over the last ten years.

The drug of choice for injecting in IDUs in these cities is Buprenorphine, and it is frequently cocktailed with sedative and anti-histaminic injections leading to venous thrombosis and abscess formation; the HIV prevalence varies from 1 per cent in IDUs of Kolkatato 31 per cent in Chennai. The reported high needle syringe sharing rate among IDUs and observed switching of large number of heroin smokers to injection drug use during heroin-drought in these cities, indicate the need for large scale intervention. Research should also be conducted to identify the factors responsible for heterogeneity in HIV prevalence among IDUs in these cities so that appropriate intervention could be designed and national response to HIV in IDUs could be augmented.

HIV epidemic in pediatric population

The latest sentinel surveillance data from ante-natal clinics in seven metro citizen the country reveal that HIV infection has crossed 2 per cent in Mumbai, is more than 1 per cent in Hyderabad, Bangalore, Chennai and below 1 per cent in Kolkata, Ahmedabad and Delhi. This clearly indicates that the cities with 1 per cent or more HIV prevalence among pregnant women have already fallen under the grip of HIV epidemic in pediatric population as well. It has also been recorded that Manipur – which had the earliest explosive HIV epidemic among IDUs – has started seeing the impact of the disease in the form of many AIDS orphans, a phenomenon which needs a very different set of interventions not yet witnessed on a large scale.

The government of India has taken commendable steps in launching hospital-based prevention of HIV transmission from pregnant mothers to children through administration of short course AZT in 11 centres located in the worst hit States. However it is worth noting that two-thirds or more of the deliveries take place at husbands' or parents' homes of the pregnant women. Moreover, stigma and discrimination often come in the way of positive women accessing health care, especially in government facilities.

A national feasibility study of administering short-term AZT intervention among HIV-infected mothers to prevent mother-to-child transmission of HIV was conducted between April 2000 and July 2001. The study was conducted from 11 medical institutes in five States (Maharashtra, Tamil Nadu, Andhra Pradesh, Karnataka and Manipur) in India. It was observed that a total of 192474 women were offered HIV counselling and testing services during the study period, of which 171471 (89 per cent) received the services.

There was a further decline in HIV test uptake; 103,681 among 171,471 (60 per cent) undertook HIV test of which 1724 (1.7 per cent) were HIV positive. Despite best possible efforts of health care providers – backed up by counselling services in the medical institutes – some of the HIV positive women in the study never came back for the test results and only 44 per cent (751/1,724) took AZT prophylaxis which was to be received from the study centres.

Willingness to deliver at the institutes was another inclusion criterion in the study that did not allow many women to enrol in the study, as they wanted to go to their parents' home in third trimester and deliver there. This further emphasises the need for innovative community-based approach for prevention of third wave of the epidemic in the pediatric population in the country. Future programme planning should look for alternate ways of reaching out to 'mothers-in-need', especially through involvement of non-government and community based organisations.

Migration

Migration has added another dimension to the epidemic in India. The country has seen – and continues to see – significant migration, both between states, and between the country and other neighbouring countries. Nepal and Bangladesh have extremely porous international borders with India. While Bangladesh still has a low HIV epidemic, the HIV prevalence among sex workers in Nepal has reached 16 per cent and among IDUs 50 per cent.

Some of the destination states of India also happen to be those registering high HIV prevalence. These include the more industrialised States of Maharashtra, Gujarat and Andhra Pradesh. These States attract male and female labourers from all over the country, but particularly from those States with lower income levels such as Uttar Pradesh, Bihar, Rajashthan and Madhya Pradesh. While these latter states have relatively low levels of reported HIV infection, labour migration to high prevalence states may soon change the scenario. Indeed many of the migrating men leave their wives and families behind, thus increasing the likelihood that they will visit sex workers during their stays away from home. Migration due to various factors such as eviction of tribal people from forests to be owned by government in Rajasthan or fatal ethnic clash in Manipur have also been documented as reasons why women are forced to take up prostitution as alternate means of living.

Blood safety

The cornerstone of programmes to reduce HIV transmission by transfusion of blood/blood product is the testing of all blood donations for HIV antibody. Although the situation has improved in India after the Supreme Court verdict in this direction, 100 per cent safe blood/blood product transfusion is yet to be achieved in India. The main issue is of supply; demand always exceeds supply and currently only 60 per cent of the demand is being met through official sources, which has serious implications for HIV transmission in the country.

States with relatively less developed rural areas and difficult hilly terrain with inadequate health care delivery services have this as a problem, but also in states such as Mumbai and West Bengal, concerns have been raised in this regard. As centralised blood transfusion services would be difficult in as vast a country as India where these are operated by government, voluntary and commercial establishments, and development of standardised processes and centralised quality assurance programmes have been recommended.

Additional inputs that could boost up the whole prevention programme in the country in this field are training of health care providers on 'rational use of blood transfusion', 'component therapy instead of whole blood transfusion' and innovative donor deferral criteria in conjunction with blood screening. While the issues discussed above may seem diverse, needing completely separate sets of interventions, there are some fundamental commonalties underlying the spread of the virus, which call out for a developmental approach to interventions. These common features can be brought out by first asking the following two questions:

— what are the factors that facilitate the spread of the virus
— where will the impact of the epidemic be felt the most

In India the major route of transmission is sexual, followed by infected blood and blood products. Taking the sexual route of transmission first, given the age structure of the population, a large majority of India's population is in the sexually active age group (49.5 per cent in the age group 15–49 as reported in

NFHS-2). This figure is about 6 per centage points higher in the urban areas than in the rural areas, indicating possibly migration. Another point to note is that all of India has an adverse sex ratio, which deteriorated further by 2001; thus there are fewer females per 1,000 males. Secondly, a slightly lower proportion of female aged 6 and above have never married compared to males.

Finally, women in India marry at much younger ages than men, and both men and women marry at younger ages in rural than in urban areas. To really understand the extent of risky behaviour of individuals, one also needs some estimates of pre-marital, extra-marital as well as sexual behaviour of never-married individuals. While these figures are not easily available, it can only be conjectured that these practices exist just like anywhere else in India as well.

In any case, these demographic facts do indicate the wide prevalence of marriage as well as the vulnerability of women in India, two facts that are very important in the context of the HIV/AIDS epidemic. It also implies that it is *possible* for this sub-population of sexually active individuals to acquire the infection, though the *probability* will depend on their specific risk behaviours. While there exists now a large amount of literature on who, why and how risky sex behaviour occurs, the simple fact is that risky sex can occur only in one of two ways: deliberately (with correct knowledge) or non-deliberately.

While no statistics exist on the proportion of each, it may be safe to conclude that most individuals have a long time horizon and will not wilfully engage in behaviour that may jeopardize his/her life. However, there are some factors that may increase even this kind of behaviour, and these factors have to do with a much shorter time horizon (i.e. they do not care too much about the future) emanating from a variety of reasons, or a lifestyle that has little to offer by way of a peaceful and stable existence. But, a majority of risk behaviour is undertaken with lack of knowledge about the implications of such behaviour. Thus we need to answer two additional questions in turn:

- Who are least likely to be informed?
- Who are most likely to have a shorter time horizon?

It is our contention that there are a number of factors that need to be considered to address these questions, and these are the commonalties that cut across risk groups and behaviour and these are indicated below:

- *Poverty*: one of the main reasons for poverty is unemployment and/or underemployment. In addition, the poor will also include seasonally employed, a large section of the informal sector workers, beggars, street children, sex workers, slum dwellers.
- Illiterate, uneducated and less educated.
- Marginalised and disempowered populations: the poor, the uneducated, women, minorities, refugees, street children, beggars, sexual minorities.
- Those with interrupted family lives either by lifestyle choice or by force of circumstances: migrants, frequent long-distance travellers, armed forces, refugees, slum dwellers.
- Women, especially those who are poor, uneducated, unemployed and generally disempowered due to the cultural and patriarchal structures of Indian society.
- The youth and the elderly, especially those belonging to any of the vulnerable groups mentioned above Many of these factors go into making a large majority of India's population *potentially* vulnerable to HIV via the sexual route of transmission.

Care and support

Historically in India, more emphasis has been given to HIV prevention. Time is however ripe that HIV/AIDS care is also discussed along with prevention. Those already infected and in advanced stages of HIV disease are in substantial number in the country; without effective case management approach with currently available antiretroviral therapy, neither prevention nor care needs will be addressed. Some important issues under care and support are women-headed and children-headed households, orphans and the elderly. There is no national structure for care and support, and in the absence of social security, insurance or other safety nets, the issue takes on an even more urgent tone.

A few organisations such as the HIV/AIDS Alliance and Naz India are filling this gap in three states of Andhra Pradesh, Tamil Nadu and Delhi through their network of implementing partner organisations. The needs include medical support, counselling, livelihood, educational support and working with the families and communities to reduce stigma and discrimination. It is being increasingly realised that care can be given at home and not necessarily in an institutional setting.

It is now necessary to focus attention on innovative ways of extending support to those affected, without injecting elements of inequity across socioeconomic classes or across disease categories. Replicable and feasible models of care and support need to be developed. One important lacuna so far in the care and support efforts have been a lack of legal framework, which ensures the rights of PLWHA, especially in the areas of workplace and health care settings.

RESPONSES

India's AIDS programmes are implemented through the National AIDS Control Organisation (NACO), a semi-independent organisation established in 1992 within the Health Ministry. Its special status was intended to prevent the bureaucratic delays that normally plague India's decision-making process.

India's National AIDS Control Policy adheres to the following strategy in its effort to prevent and control HIV/AIDS throughout the country:

i) Prevent the further spread of the disease by:
   - Improving HIV/AIDS awareness and providing people with the necessary tools to protect themselves;
   - Controlling sexually transmitted infections and promoting condom use; and
   - Ensuring the availability of safe blood and blood products.

ii) Create a socioeconomic environment that enables individuals to protect themselves from infection and allows families and communities to provide care and support to people living with HIV/AIDS.

iii) Improve services—both in hospitals and through community-based home care—that provide care for people living with HIV/AIDS.

The National AIDS Control Organisation, with financial assistance from the World Bank, is currently implementing the second phase of its National AIDS Control Programme. The objectives of this phase are to:

- Reduce the spread of HIV infection in at-risk populations;
- Reduce the spread of HIV in the general population;
- Strengthen the impact and sustainability of national, state, and local HIV/AIDS programmes;
- Build capacity to provide low-cost, community-based care; and
- Promote intersectoral links to combat HIV/AIDS.

NACO put froward a the National AIDS Control Programme (NACP) – a fully centrally-sponsored scheme – which comprises Surveillance, Programme Management, Information, Education and Communication (IEC), Blood Safety, Condom Promotion, Control of STDs, and Clinical Management. Needless to say, much less was known about the determinants and outcome of HIV/AIDS at that point than is known now.

This first phase (1992–1999) of the project was mainly to be financed by a Government of India contribution of $14.1 million, an IDA credit of $84 million and a WHO co-financing grant of $1.5 million. It should be noted that the GOI contribution was actually much higher than the original estimate and came to $27.5 million. In addition, there were two important additional sources of financing: USAID and DFID. Now, in Phase 2 of the NACP, the objectives of NACO continue to be similar; these are:

— To reduce spread of HIV infection.
— To strengthen India's capacity to respond to HIV/AIDS on a long-term basis.

The targets envisaged in the NACP-2 are the following:

— Reduce blood-borne transmission of HIV to less than 1 per cent of total transmissions.
— To introduce Hepatitis C as the fifth mandatory test for blood screening.
— To set up new and upgrade existing blood banks as well blood component separation units.
— To attain awareness level of at least 90 per cent among youth and those in reproductive ages.
— Training of NGOs for targeted intervention programmes among high risk groups, to in turn promote condom use to at least 90 per cent in these groups.
— Conduct annual Family Health Awareness Campaigns among general population; provision of drugs for control of STDs and RTIs.
— Promotion of voluntary testing facilities so that every district in the country will have at least one voluntary testing facility.
— Use of interactive awareness campaigns like folk arts and street theatre.

— Cover all the schools and universities under awareness programmes.

— Promote organisations of PLWHA and give then financial support to form self-help groups The above are firm targets that the NACP-II hopes to achieve by the end of 2004. Further, the major components of NACP-II under which these targets would be achieved are:

  — *Priority targeted interventions for high risk population*: this has to be done mainly through NGOs/CBOs/Public sector.

  — *Preventive interventions for the general population:* this has to be done through IEC, awareness campaigns, voluntary testing and counselling (VTC), reduction of transmission by infected blood and blood products and prevention of occupational exposure.

  — *Low cost care for people living with HIV/AIDS*: financial and technical assistance to be provided to states/UTs for home-based and community-based care.

  — Institutional strengthening, including strengthening surveillance activities and research and development.

  — *Inter-sectoral collaboration:* coordination within the Ministry of Health and Family Welfare, as well as other central ministries.

The main emphasis on NACP-II is on clean and adequate supply of blood, IEC and targeted interventions among high-risk groups. The achievements of the first phase however lie in responding swiftly, building programme capacity, efforts to tone up the surveillance system, getting the blood banks to supply cleaner blood and raising awareness. A major innovation in Phase I of NACP was the replacement of the earlier structure of State AIDS Cell by State AIDS Control Society. This step was taken to ensure easier disbursement of funds, lack of delays and more decentralisation in decisionmaking. The other has been to move from developing and disseminating IEC materials to actually translating these into action by using the targeted intervention approach.

Table 2 below gives a break-up of the Phase II outlay by major areas of focus. As the table indicates, prevention among low-risk groups is to receive the highest allocation (33.7 per cent), followed by institutional strengthening and prevention among high-risk groups (24.8 per cent and 23 per cent respectively).

Table 2. Allocation of funds for NACP-II

Components	*Outlay (Rs. Crores)*	*Per centage*
Prevention among high-risk groups	265.6	23.0
Prevention among low-risk groups	389.1	33.7
Care of HIV/AIDS	163.3	14.1
Institutional strengthening	286.5	24.8
Intersectoral collaboration	50.6	4.4
Total	1155.1	100.0
USAID – AVERT project	166	–
DFID	104	–

Out of the total Rs. 1155.1 crores in the NACP- II, World Bank has provided Rs. 959.1 crores; the remaining Rs. 196 crores is to be provided by the Government of India. In other words, the World Bank is to provide 83 per cent of the proposed outlay for NACP-II. In addition to these two sources of funding, the two other major sources of funding are USAID and DFID. The USAID has extended support of Rs. 166 crores, to the Government of Maharashtra for implementation of AVERT project, based on the earlier success of the still on-going APAC project in Tamil Nadu. DFID has given assistance of Rs. 104 crores, for Sexual Health projects in the states of Andhra Pradesh, Gujarat, Kerala and Orissa

The overall focus of the NACP is towards prevention and control: about 60 per cent of its funds are allocated to prevent the transmission of HIV. Also, the other major partners – DFID and USAID – are also heavily involved in prevention. Care and support receive a much smaller allocation – 14 per cent – in the programme. In fact, the number of Targeted Interventions

(TI) projects in India are 475, with the highest numbers being carried out in Tamil Nadu, followed by Maharashtra. DFID and USAID as mentioned above fund many of these.

It is interesting to note that there are no NACP-funded TI projects in the following states and UTs: Andaman & Nicobar Islands, Bihar, Dadra and Nagar Haveli, Daman and Diu, Delhi, Jammu and Kashmir, Lakshwadeep, Meghalaya, Pondicherry, Sikkim and Uttar Pradesh. However, it is also true that there are instances of non-governmental organisations running targeted interventions in different states; for example, there is an EU-funded 5-city oral sublingual buprenorphine substitution programme for IDUs, which includes Delhi.

International Help and Donor Interventions

Organisations involved in both prevention and control programmes as well as care and support can be divided into four categories: the UN agencies, bilaterals, international NGOs (INGOs) and domestic NGOs/CBOs.

UN agencies

USAID is one of the largest donors to HIV/AIDS prevention and control programmes in the country, allocating $12.2 in 2002, an increase from $9 million in 2001. USAID/India's primary objective is to focus on HIV prevention and containment of the epidemic. Prevention activities target at-risk populations, such as commercial sex workers and truck drivers, who are likely core transmitters of HIV in India. However, USAID/India is also working to build awareness in low-risk rural populations and will endeavour to promote prevention activities through health services outreach projects., USAID bilateral assistance is focused in Tamil Nadu and Maharashtra, states with adult prevalence greater than 1 per cent.

USAID has developed a partnership approach with the Government of India, non-governmental organisations, businesses, and others to fight HIV. Emphasis is placed on community-based and work-based approaches to controlling the epidemic. USAID began to tackle India's HIV/AIDS epidemic in 1992 with the development of the AIDS Prevention and Control (APAC) project in the southern Indian state of Tamil Nadu, one of India's recognised epicentres.

In 1999, USAID expanded its programme to include the state of Maharashtra, where antenatal HIV prevalence is approaching 2 per cent. The seven-year, $41.5 million AVERT activity funds comprehensive prevention and care programmes throughout the state of Maharashtra. The major activities under both projects include financial and technical assistance to non-governmental organisations to undertake targeted interventions on HIV/AIDS, capacity building of health care providers, and behaviour change communication, including mass media, condom promotion, sexually transmitted infection prevention, and advocacy.

In 2002, USAID increased the number of grants to nongovernmental organisations, and began addressing new issues such as care and support for HIV-infected persons, voluntary counselling and testing, interventions with industrial workers, and geographic expansion of the APAC project to include Pondicherry, an adjacent and culturally similar area to the present activity area in Tamil Nadu.

Other USAID-funded HIV/AIDS activities include supporting the National Ports project, Project Lighthouse. Implemented by Population Services International in the 12 major ports of India, this project addresses vulnerable populations associated with ports, which include casual workers, migrants, formal port employees, truckers, and commercial sex workers. The project strategies include behaviour change communication, condom promotion, and sexually transmitted infection treatment.

USAID also supports Family Health International through the IMPACT project. Family Health International supports nongovernmental organisations to provide support to children infected and affected by HIV/AIDS and other vulnerable children, pilot activities on care and support, applied research and developing models for HIV/AIDS programming.

Additional USAID-supported activities include the following:

i) *Capacity building:* The Mission supports the National AIDS Control Organisation by providing financial and technical assistance to national programmes. USAID also provides grants to medical colleges and institutions to improve HIV/AIDS and sexually transmitted infection training for health care providers.

ii) *Prevention*: The 10-year, $10 million AIDS Prevention and Control project in Tamil Nadu supports non-governmental organisation efforts to design and implement community-based prevention programmes that target at-risk populations, such as sex workers and their clients, patients with sexually transmitted infections, slum dwellers, and truckers and their helpers. The project emphasises preventive behaviour through peer education, the promotion of condoms, and improved treatment of sexually transmitted infections.

   The AVERT project in Maharashtra state supports prevention efforts in urban and peri-urban areas and works to increase the role of non-governmental organisations in HIV prevention.

iii) *Care and support*: Through both the bilateral and field support programmes, USAID is exploring innovative models for care and support, including home and community-based care.

iv) *Protection of children affected by AIDS:* USAID supports comprehensive projects addressing the special needs of children both infected and affected by HIV/AIDS throughout the country.

v) *Condoms:* To expand and improve condom distribution, USAID-supported projects provide financial support and technical assistance to the commercial sector. The programme assists the Drug Controller of India in strengthening quality control and monitoring activities, and is working with manufacturers to improve condom packaging. The programme also supports the private and commercial sectors in creating new diagnostic products and improving the quality and marketing of existing products.

vi) *Research and surveillance*: USAID funds annual HIV risk-behavioural surveillance surveys that track key behaviour changes, such as condom use, treatment-seeking of sexually transmitted infections, and decreases in sexual contacts with non-regular partners. In Tamil Nadu, behavioural surveillance surveys and available seroprevalence data suggest a promising trend in that state: an increase in HIV prevention behaviour and a decrease in HIV prevalence levels. Additional clinical research activities are being planned through IndiaCLEN.

Bilaterals, Private Foundations and international NGOs

The major bilateral players are USAID, DFID, CIDA, Sida and AusAID. European Union (EU) has also emerged as an important player. Besides these, there are other international Foundations and NGOs (INGOs) like the Ford Foundation, MacArthur Foundation, Population Council, Family Health International (FHI), HIV/AIDS Alliance etc. that have added significance to the overall activities around HIV/AIDS in India.

Most of the donor interventions are in the areas of prevention through targeted interventions and awareness campaigns, and primarily focused in the states of Maharashtra, Andhra Pradesh, Tamil Nadu, Manipur, West Bengal, Kerala and Gujarat. One of the few international agencies working on HIV/AIDS care and support in India is Oxfam in Manipur and India HIV/AIDS Alliance in the states of Andhra Pradesh, Tamil Nadu and Delhi. The states with limited donor HIV/AIDS interventions are Bihar, Rajasthan, Karnataka, Orissa, Assam, Arunachal Pradesh and Tripura. Many of these states are also underdeveloped with high levels of poverty, as discussed in the first section.

Some of the other international organisations that are working on HIV/AIDS in India are CARE India who are in the process of negotiating a US $ 15–20 million grant (from USAID) to work in seven low prevalent states across the country. Their focus will be on prevention and awareness building amongst vulnerable groups. BBC World Service Trust is working on communication for the northern states of Uttar Pradesh, Rajasthan and Delhi. Catholic Relief Services, Plan International, Action AID, World Vision are other international organisations also working on HIV/AIDS who are beginning to support more prevention as well as care and support programmes in the high prevalent states.

CEDPA will be working on HIV/AIDS and youth as a part of the USAID funded IFPS project in Uttar Pradesh. Some of the other Foundations funding in India are Bill and Melinda Gates Foundation (for whom India and HIV/AIDS are becoming a key focus area), Packard Foundation (focus on Bihar and Jharkhand for reproductive health and sexuality), Francois Xavier Bagnoud (FXB), Elton John Foundation, Richard Gere Foundation, etc.

National NGOs

In addition to these organisations mentioned above, India has seen an emergence of several competent NGOs who have often filled in the gaps left by other players, especially in working with vulnerable groups. While it is difficult to list all the NGOs working in India on HIV/AIDS and related issues, some of the more notable ones are Y.R.G. Care (Chennai), Indian Network of Positive People (INP+), Naz Foundation India Trust (Delhi), Sahara (Delhi), Sharan (Delhi), SPARSHA (Society for Positive Atmosphere and Related Support to HIV/AIDS, Kolkata), Freedom Foundation (Bangalore, Hyderabad), SOS Medical Foundation (Nasik), Prayas (Pune), Sangram (Sangli), CASA (Mumbai), Prepare (Chennai), Lawyers Collective (Mumbai and Delhi), Durbar Mahila Samanvaya Committee (DMSC, Kolkata) etc. In addition to these, India has seen the emergence of several NGO conglomerations such as FINGODAP, working on drug and AIDS, and India Network of NGOs (INN).

The rich NGO experience unfortunately has not been adequately analysed, evaluated and documented, including showcasing of best practices. This has meant that this resource has been both nonscalable as well as underutilised. This remains an important area where donors can step in to facilitate a wider dissemination and utilisation of knowledge, experience and best practices emanating from the NGO/CBO sector. Also, the NGOs often lack technical as well as administrative capacities, and have very little knowledge or understanding of research. The donors can help by lending technical support as well as research support to these organisations.

India HIV/AIDS Alliance

The India HIV/AIDS Alliance has been primarily focusing on care and support programmemes in the states of Andhra Pradesh, Tamil Nadu and Delhi. The purpose has been to provide people living with HIV/AIDS (PLHA), children affected by AIDS (CAA) and their families with appropriate and adequate support in their clinical and psychosocial needs through the delivery of integrated home and community care by NGOs/CBOs; and to strengthen communities in their response to the epidemic and the mitigation of its impact.

The major lessons learned from the implementation experience have been that integrated community development organisations are more flexible and innovative in identifying and planning community based care and support activities, and also address stigma and discrimination, in comparison to those that have existing institutional services or are involved in prevention through targeted interventions. These organisations also address sustainability issues early on in project development. Participatory Community Assessment (PCA) and use of participatory tools is also a good start up activity for implementation of HIV/AIDS care and support projects.

Project Concern International (PCI)

Project Concern International (PCI) has been working on HIV/AIDS in India for the last few years. The major focus of their HIV/AIDS interventions has been behaviour change through counselling and education, condom promotion, STI treatment and counselling (syndromic management of STIs), training on STIs, HIV/AIDS and sex and sexuality. The special groups for focus are truckers, street and working children, PLHA and their families, sex workers, injecting drug users, adolescents and *devadasis*. Their HIV/AIDS care and support interventions have included home based care and support for PLHA through medical and psychosocial care, training and orientation of PLHA, their families and community members.

PCI has provided a forum for NGOs to come together for discussions and experience sharing that has been beneficial for cross fertilisation of ideas and innovative intervention development. Implementation of Management Information Systems (MIS) for the partner NGOs as also financial systems that are capable of capturing information on local donation, cost recovery mechanisms, income-generating projects and community contributions have greatly enhanced the effective functioning of these NGOs.

APAC/VHS/USAID

AIDS Prevention and Control (APAC) project is administered by Voluntary Health Services (VHS), Chennai, with financial assistance from USAID, under a bilateral agreement with the Government of India. APAC initiated HIV/AIDS prevention in Tamil Nadu in the year 1996 with the overall goal of reducing the sexual transmission of HIV in the state. The project supports NGO partners to implement thematic intervention projects reaching "Truckers and Helpers", "Women in Prostitution", "People Living in Slums" and tourists. It also conducts HIV Behaviour Surveillance Survey (BSS) to capture the intervention efforts, and to inform the intervention programme. Altogether five rounds of BSS have been completed by now.

APAC is the only project in India that has attempted to systematically look into the changes in risk behaviour of different population groups since 1996 through 2000, and has used the behaviour surveillance data for informing interventions. The experience of APAC for tripartite collaboration and documented behaviour change are certainly worth emulating after adapting to different local conditions.

Department for International Development (DFID)

DFID has been implementing the Sexual Health Project in West Bengal with the focus of HIV/AIDS control programmes and developing IEC techniques. DFID has also supported a national Healthy Highways Project with the truckers' community. The pilot project has been integrated into the NACPII. In addition, DFID has formulated "partnership for sexual health" projects for the prevention and control of HIV/AIDS and other sexually transmitted infections in the states of Andhra Pradesh, Gujarat, Kerala and Orissa. The objectives of the project are:

i) To ensure better sexual health for people vulnerable to sexually transmitted diseases (STDs) and HIV, especially the poor; and

ii) lowering incidence of sexually transmitted infections in the four states. The components of the project are:

   a) surveillance,

   b) condom programming by ensuring that quality condoms are made available and acceptable to those who are vulnerable to STDs/HIV through effective social marketing,

   c) strengthening service providers to respond to clients needs through targeted interventions for vulnerable groups, such as sex workers and their clients, men having sex with men, migrant workers and prison inmates.

Some of the lessons learned are: political will is the essence of success of HIV/AIDS prevention programs; establishing and maintaining decision making systems needs full co-operation from the government; planning for HIV/AIDS prevention programmes at the state level needs greater co-ordination between GO-NGO; having a Management Agency makes co-ordination feasible; collating the strengths of each organisation is the key to success; build capacities of the states to sustain the programme which includes developing local expertise in HIV/AIDS prevention.

Role of Private Sector

In addition to the government and national and international donors and NGOs, the private sector in India has also made its presence felt in HIV prevention activities, especially around issues like workplace interventions, community programmes and support to NGOs. The Confederation of Indian Industry (CII) has supported over 1700 companies in establishing workplace programmes and has provided income generation opportunities for people living with HIV/AIDS.

B Muthuraman, the managing director of Tata Steel, in his statement on the HIV(+) and AIDS Policy on 1 October, 2001 mentioned that Tata Steel would take measures to prevent the incidence and spread of HIV and AIDS in the society. In case of need, the company would arrange to provide counselling and medical guidance to these patients and their families. AIDS awareness and treatment of drug dependence are two other related issues that TATA has been concerned for quite some time now.

Since mid-'1990s Tata Steel has been providing infrastructure support for running drug detoxification centre in Barandi, Bihar where its collaborating partner organisation 'The Calcutta Samaritans' is in-charge of the technical inputs as well as service provision. The changing scenario of drug use from heroin smoking to synthetic pharmaceutical injecting among the local youths including a few industrial workers in and around Jamshedpur called for such an action and the present status of this collaboration exemplifies a successful networking between private corporate sector and NGO, many of which kind should take place within the country in order to achieve a significant public health impact on HIV/AIDS prevention and care.

Other examples of such activities include Tata Tea's collaboration with tea plantation workers in Kerala. Similar collaboration and business coalitions against HIV/AIDS are being set up in different states, and CII has also set up the Indian Business Trust for HIV/AIDS. In another example of donors collaborating with the private sector, the ILO in consultation with its Indian tripartite constituents and NACO has developed a three-phased programme, aimed at establishing a sustainable national action on HIV/AIDS prevention, care and support in the world of work.

The notable features of the ILO project include: guidance to the project by a high-level project management team, mobilisation of partners through stakeholders meetings and consultations/seminars, etc., in an attempt to put HIV/AIDS on the agenda, research based advocacy, documentation of corporate responses to HIV/AIDS, compilation and dissemination of existing research studies on HIV/AIDS in the world of work, initiation of action research projects and capacity building.

EVIDENCE-BASED INTERVENTIONS

From the point of view of the national response, the main strengths of NACP in India have been the following:

- swiftness of response
- setting up a fairly strong organisation like the NACO
- ability to procure in two stages a high level of funding commitment from a major organisation like the World Bank

— ability to build up state level capacities
— ability to attract additional donors and their funding
— successful collaboration with major bilaterals and INGOs
— ability to work with Indian NGOs

Gaps, however, remain even today in the NACP as well as in the non-government response. Most of these gaps have been recognised, but there has been an inability to deal effectively with these, mainly because of an imperfect understanding of how to move forward.

Below we list some of the continued problems despite over a decade-long response:

— Inability to integrate HIV/AIDS into the mainstream of public health activities
— Inability to reduce stigma and discrimination
— Inadequate focus on vulnerability factors, especially poverty, illiteracy and disempowerment
— Inadequate geographic and population coverage in terms of targeted interventions
— Inadequate focus on care and support
— Inadequate attention paid to the issues around antiretroviral treatment
— Lack of focus on generating evidence, especially around risk practices and treatment-seeking behaviour among bridge population and core transmitters.
— Almost complete neglect of monitoring and evaluation of programmes

Of these, the most damaging have been the first and the last one. It is our contention that by making HIV/AIDS a stand-alone and vertical programme, which is not integrated into an overall public health framework, we may have added to the stigma and discrimination surrounding it. The high-profile activities and funding have also brought out in sharp focus the possible inequities that such programmes might inject into both national health policy as well as overall welfare policies. This is because, it is not always clear why HIV/AIDS should merit greater attention than other infectious diseases, or why those who are infected should merit greater assistance than those who are not infected but fatally sick.

This inadequate recognition given to equity issues has been instrumental in bringing criticism to the extent that some have questioned the very need for such a high-funded project for AIDS. In addition to not adequately recognising the need for integration into other health programmes right at the outset, or even midway into the first phase, the problem was compounded by messages of IEC that made HIV and AIDS stand out like some frightening and severe malady, which happens only to those who ask for it by behaving in manners not consistent with Indian morals.

To a great extent, this high profiling of the epidemic was also due to the multiplicity of players, especially the international donor communities, which poured funding into prevention and control activities. A related and equally important point is that while much of the NACO core funds as well as co-financing went into prevention and control, almost no mechanism was put in place to evaluate these prevention activities. A prime example is IEC, which has often been implemented through targeted interventions aimed at high-risk population.

There is no allocation made in the NACP budget for monitoring and evaluation. While additional funding is always welcome in a cash-strapped country, funding does not seem to be the problem in India. It is an imperfect and inadequate understanding of what works, which can come only if evaluation procedures are put in place before activities are being planned. Evaluation is a scientific process and cannot generally be done well in an ex-post fashion. Another example is the proposed scaling up of the MTCT programme, which has been put in place before any evaluation of the current programme, has been done.

Unfortunately, the other donors have also not insisted in scientific evaluations, though it is being recognised now that there is a need to know whether good money is being thrown after bad programmes. As for care and support, it is clear that no single organisation or even the government can shoulder the care responsibilities of AIDS patients; it is neither feasible nor is it equitable in terms of other diseases.

However, it is possible to remove the constraints in care-seeking and patient-management with careful planning, and helping groups to help themselves in planning for the future. This would, of course, require a completely new and truly developmental approach to the epidemic, requiring integration of poverty reduction and other welfare programmes into HIV/AIDS activities. This is again not something that has been attempted in any serious fashion.

As for the national NGOs, while there are many that are doing commendable work, there is a lot going on that is not being evaluated either. If national and large donor-driven programmes are not evaluated, this is even truer of NGO activities in India. There is no monitoring and evaluation at all, especially outcome evaluation. While figures are not easily available, it is probably true that much of the funding continues to flow into behaviour change and IEC activities – an area where it is easy to put in money, but which is difficult to evaluate in terms of outcome.

On the other hand, national NGOs, including some international ones with branches in India are also filling in one important gap in response – care. There are now a few NGOs and INGOs like YRG Care, Naz Foundation – India Trust, HIV AIDS Alliance, ARCON etc., that are catering to the needs of at least a small proportion of PLWHAs. Finally, in all the programmes — national or international —there has been a lack of research component, operational or otherwise. Except for some organisations like Voluntary Health Services (VHS), NGOs and INGOs have almost never undertaken serious research into areas of their interventions. One aspect of this omission has meant that there has been an imperfect understanding of the impact of the epidemic on different sectors. The one that should concern India immediately is the health sector.

There is almost no research that looks into the impact that increased morbidity and mortality will have on the health sector in India. There are some studies however on the impact on individuals and households, though these results have not been put to much use. All this implies that policymakers have no channels of being informed about what is needed, where and how.

Scaling up of Intervention

While the prevalence of HIV in India may seem relatively low – 0.7 per cent of the general adult population compared with rates of over 20 per cent in South Africa, Zimbabwe and Botswana – the infection has now been detected in all the states and union territories. It is no longer confined to vulnerable groups such as sex workers and transport workers, or to urban areas, and here lies the necessity for urgent scaled up responses for prevention of further spread of HIV. Pilot HIV intervention projects supported by different donor agencies during phase-I of the National AIDS Control Programme (NACP) in India have identified a number of essential elements of intervention, which were incorporated in the second phase of programme planning.

However, it is important to understand that while there are some essential elements (involvement of communities, creation of enabling environment, peer-based behaviour change intervention etc) that go into any intervention, each context and setting is different, and therefore scaling up should be done with great caution. In other words, exactly the same "best practice" – for example Sonagachi sex worker intervention – when put in another setting with all the essential elements in place may not yield the same outcomes.

There may be a number of reasons why scaling-up and replication has not happened – even for some of the best practices. While a few such practices have been documented, inadequate attention has been paid to producing a complete blue print of these interventions. To do so, attention will have to be paid to:

(a) context; for example, power brokers in a sex work setting,
(b) capacity building of community members,
(c) how community members can be engaged in planning, implementation and evaluation.

There are several interventions carried out by a multiplicity of agencies and organisations all over India. However, there has been very little documentation of these interventions. Without mapping the universal set of interventions, it is not possible to take the next step of evaluating which of these actually work.

Generation of Evidence

Inadequate current response to HIV/AIDS in India stems from the fact that the knowledge base about the epidemic is far from perfect. There are some critical gaps in information with regard to:

— HIV/STD Surveillance in female sex workers, low risk male population groups and migrant labourers
— Countrywide mapping of HIV/AIDS interventions in prevention as well as care and support
— Treatment seeking behaviour of vulnerable groups such as sex workers and IDUs
— Risk practices and treatment seeking behaviour of bridge population
— Socio-economic impact on households, various sectors especially the health sector and the economy as a whole
— Cost-effectiveness of interventions

For informed and effective policymaking, it is imperative to start generating evidence in these areas. The information can be generated by a wide variety of organisations and by using various methods, including operations research. It must be pointed out here that good research on the epidemic must always be based on the involvement of individuals affected by HIV.

CONCLUSIONS AND RECOMMENDATIONS ON PRIORITIES

India has been able to respond fairly quickly and comprehensively to the AIDS epidemic. However, there are still many areas where more focus and attention are required. The main lacunae in the current collective response has been that despite a recognition of the need to mainstream, strategies of poverty reduction and prevention and control and care and support have remained more or less parallel.

Thus, the Planning Commission of the country has yet to take a serious note of the epidemic and the need for integrating responses with other developmental ones. This lack of mainstreaming has also resulted in a paradoxical situation, where too much visibility accorded to HIV/AIDS has added to the stigma and discrimination by creating a mysterious world around the epidemic. This could be eliminated or at least reduced only by an approach which recognises that for successful prevention and control it is essential to pay attention to vulnerability factors, especially poverty, illiteracy and disempowerment.

The other shortfall of the current response is the geographic gaps that exist in prevention and control measures; while some states and areas have received a lot of focus, others have received very little. Thus, for instance, some of the most underdeveloped states like Orissa and Bihar have very little happening there compared to states like Tamil Nadu and Maharashtra. The low prevalence in these states is absolutely misleading because of the many vulnerability factors that make them potentially susceptible to high rates of transmission.

Another feature of the current response is the almost complete omission of monitoring and evaluation of programmes; there are very few interventions that have been accompanied by evaluation to see whether these work and to what extent. This is potentially a worrying situation since resources are scarce, and there is the danger that more resources will be spent on programmes that do not work very well.

In general there has been a lack of focus on generating evidence, especially around risk practices and treatment-seeking behaviour among bridge population and core transmitters. There is therefore the need to compile best practices in different types of interventions, from the point of view of scalability. Based on these conclusions, we present the recommendations and priorities below.

General priorities

i) *Emphasis on both prevention and control as well as care and support*: the epidemic has been around for more than 15 years now in India. But infections continue to occur in new areas and new groups, clearly indicating the need for continued efforts on prevention. At the same time, the need for care and support of those affected has increased enormously. Therefore donors should still treat prevention as their primary focus. At the same time, it should increasingly try to find innovative ways of dealing with issues of care and support.

ii) *Scaling up*: the following are essential components that need focus before scaling up.

- — mapping of interventions across the country
- — analysis and documentation of what works
- — estimation of size of vulnerable groups, especially overlooked groups like unorganised sex workers in cabin-restaurants
- — constraints faced in increasing coverage through scaled up responses

iii) *Priorities under prevention*: these are some of the key issues that need to be considered

- *Low risk population*: situational analysis, operational research and interventions for the following groups – clients of sex workers, spouse of IDUs, migrant labourers and slum population
- *Bridge population*: determinants of risk-taking behaviour and treatment seeking behaviour of bridge populations like truck drivers. Innovative ways of reaching out to these groups.
- *Informal and unorganised sector workers*: collaboration and cooperation with the private corporate sector to bring these hard-to-reach workers under the umbrella of prevention.
- *Third wave of HIV among pediatric population*: design appropriate interventions based on evidence from feasibility study that indicates reasons why most of the mothers do not access institution based interventions.
- *Cross border*: cross country collaboration to address vulnerability issues of migrant population and girls engaged in prostitution, between India and neighbouring countries like Nepal and Bangladesh.
- *Adolescents and youth*: situation analysis, operational research and appropriate interventions for this group.
- *Capacity building for effective transfusion services*: innovative blood donor deferral and training of health care providers for rational use of blood transfusion as well as component therapy, as opposed to whole blood transfusion.

iv) *Priorities under care and support*: very little is known about how best to carry out care and support programmes. Thus, the following are identified areas:

- research on socioeconomic impact, especially for households and communities, including quality and accessibility of antiretroviral therapy, and exploring mechanisms like health insurance to support increased health expenditure.

— how to foster involvement of people living with HIV/AIDS and their friends.

— Models for best practices in care and support, including costing.

v) *Research needs*: there is a need to document good research as well as support research for generating knowledge. Such research can be used by funding agencies including NACO to inform policy.

Some of the areas of research are:

— Links between poverty and other developmental factors on the one hand and HIV/AIDS on the other: this will enable answering questions like who needs what type of help, and how. The priority areas mentioned under prevention are also areas of research that can be focused upon.

vi) Impact of morbidity and mortality on the health sector: Implications for the dual epidemic of HIV and TB in India: monitoring of trend of resistance in isolates of *mycobacterium tuberculosis*.

vii) *Geographic focus*: focus on areas/states that have received little attention so far from government and other donors/NGOs.

— Need to extend analysis and coverage of areas that see out-migration to high-prevalence states in India, for example Bihar and Orissa are prime examples of neglected but vulnerable states.

— Diffusion of injection drug use in metropolitan cities of India and heterogeneity in HIV prevalence in IDUs.

viii) Monitoring and evaluation (M & E)

— Strengthen capacity for M & E of programmes and projects

— Advocacy for M & E activities
— Training in-house as well as outside on M & E.
— Lend technical support on M & E to NACO as well as other donors

ix) *Capacity building*: stress should be placed on involving communities infected and affected by HIV/AIDS
   — Roadmap for peer outreach intervention
   — Training to build capacity for operational research
   — Enhancing research and analysis capacities of NGOs as well as private corporate sector.
   — Training, orientation and sensitisation of personnel of concerned ministries and departments, such as health, home, education, labour, industry etc. This will also enhance inter-sectoral collaboration.

REFERENCES

Gupta, Indrani. "Socio-economic impact of HIV/AIDS on Individuals: A Planning Perspective from India". In *The Looming Epidemic: the Impact of HIV and AIDS in India* (ed.), Peter Godwin, Mosaic, 1998.

Indrani, "The AIDS Epidemic and the Economic Burden of Treatment in India", Presented at the Meeting of the UNAIDS Reference Group on Economics, Cuernavaca, Mexico, February 2001.

______________, Panda Samiran, Motihar Renuka, "HIV/AIDS and Development in India", Background Study for the Swedish Country Strategy for India 2003–2007, Sida, New Delhi, 2003.

Indian Council of Medical Research (ICMR), 1988, "Changing trends in sero-surveillance for HIV infection", *ICMR Bulletin* 18: 39.

Jain K., *Tribal sex seller women and HIV/AIDS infection in India. Xth International conference on AIDS*, Yokohama, Japan, 1994.

Jana S., Bandyopadhyay N., Mukherjee S., Dutta N., Basu I., Saha A., "SID/HIV intervention with sex workers in West Bengal, India", *AIDS* 1998.

Kumar M.S., Mudaliar, S., Thayagarajan, S.P., Kumar S., Selvanayagam A., "Rapid assessment and response to injecting drug use in Madras, South India", *International Journal of Drug Policy*, 11, 1–2: pp 83–98, 2002.

MAP, *The status and trends of HIV/AIDS/STI epidemics in Asia and the Pacific,* October 4 2001, Melbourne, Australia.

National AIDS Control Organisation, *Combating HIV/AIDS in India, 2000–2001*, Ministry of Health and Family Welfare. National AIDS Control Organisation, Government of India.

National Family Health Survey –2 (1998–1999), International Institute of Population Sciences. Mumbai.

Panda S., Bijaya L., Devi, N.S., et al., "Interface between drug use and sex work in Manipur, *National Medical Journal of India.* Vol 14: No 4, 2001.

Panda, S., etal., "HIV, hepatitis B and sexual practice in the street-recruited injecting drug users of Calcutta: risk perception versus observed risks", *International Journal STD & AIDS*, April, 9(4): 214–218, 1998.

Ramasundaram S., "Can India avoid being devastated by HIV", *British Medical Journal,* 324: 182–183 (26 January), 2002.

Reid G., Costigan G., *Revisiting 'The Hidden Epidemic': A Situation Assessment of Drug Use in Asia in the context of HIV/AIDS*, The Centre for Harm Reduction, The Burnet Institute, Australia. January 2002.

Salunke, S.R., Shaukat M., Hira S.K., Jagtap, M.R., "HIV/AIDS in India: A country responds to a challenge", *AIDS*; 12 (Suppl B), 1998.

Suniti Solomon, et.al., "HIV in India", *Special Contribution*, Volume 10 Issue 3 July/August 2002.

Third International Conference on AIDS INDIA, Chennai, India, December 1–5, 2001.

Times of India, State orders HIV infection enquiry at blood banks, (Kolkata) 5 March, 2002.

UNAIDS, *Workplan- 1999–2001. A Strategic Response to the HIV epidemic by the government of India, the UN and its development partners in India.*

UNAIDS/WHO, *AIDS Epidemic Update*, December 2001.

UNICEF/UNAIDS, *South Asia: The HIV/AIDS Epidemic*, 2001.

World Bank, *Confronting AIDS: Public Priorities in a Global Epidemic*, 1997.

______________, "India: New Directions in Health Sector Development at the State level: An operational perspective", *Report No. 15753-IN.* 1997.

Biblography

Alexander P., "Contextual risk versus behaviour: The impact of the legal, social and economic context of sex work on individual risk taking", *Research for Sex Work*; 4, Amsterdam, 2001

Auvert B, et al., "Ecological and individual level analysis of risk factors for HIV infection in four urban populations in sub-Saharan Africa with different levels of HIV infection", *AIDS*; 15: S15–30, 2001.

Bloom D. et al., *Health, wealth, AIDS and Poverty*, Cambridge: Harvard School of Public Health, 2002.

Bloom, S.S., et al., "Looking for change in response to the AIDS epidemic: Trends in AIDS knowledge and sexual behaviour in Zambia, 1990 through 1998", *Journal of Acquired Immune Deficiency Syndromes*; 25(1): 77–85.

Bollinger L., Stover J., *The Economic Impact of AIDS*, Washington: The Futures Group International, 1999.

Brahmbhatt H., Kigozi G., Wabwire-Mangen F. Serwadda D, Sewakambo N et al. "The effects of placental malaria on mother-to-child transmission in Rakai", Uganda. *AIDS* 2003;17:2539-2541.

Burrows D, Landman W., "Harm reduction: A key component of fighting AIDS in Russia", *Sexual Health Exchange* 2001-2; p. 5–7., 2002.

Carrasco E., "Access to Treatment as a Right to Life and Health", *Canadian HIV and AIDS Policy Law Review*; 5: 4, 2000.

Centers for Disease Control and Prevention, *Need for Sustained HIV Prevention for Gay and Bisexual Men: HIV Infections Continue at High Levels among Men of All Races with Dramatic Impact among Men of Color*, Atlanta: National Center for HIV, STD and TB Prevention, 2000.

Centers for Disease Control, "Perspectives in disease prevention and health promotion update: Universal precautions for prevention of transmission of human immunodeficiency virus, hepatitis B virus, and other pathogens in health-care settings", *MMWR Morb Mortal Wkly* Rep 1988; 37(24): 377-88.

Charter of the United Nations (VII), New York: United Nations; 1994; p. 22-8.

Cohen, D., *Mainstreaming the policy and programming response to the HIV epidemic*, New York, UNDP, 2000.

Coombe, C., *Managing the impact of HIV/AIDS on the education sector*, University of Pretoria: Centre for the study of AIDS, 2000.

Crofts N., et al., "Harm Reduction in Asia: A successful response to hidden epidemics", *AIDS*; 12 (supplement B): S109–S115, 1998.

Delor F, Hubert M., "Revisiting the concept of 'vulnerability'", *Social Science & Medicine*; 50: 1557–1570, 2000.

Desmond C., Michael K, Gow J., *The Hidden Battle: HIV/AIDS in the Family and Community*, Health Economics and HIV/AIDS Research Division (HEARD). Durban: University of Natal, 2001.

Dodds J., et al., "Increase in high-risk sexual behaviour among homosexual men", London 1996–8: crosssectional, questionnaire study, *British Medical Journal*; 320: 1510–1511, 2001.

Downing R.G., Otten, R.A., Marum E., et al.. "Optimising the delivery of HIV counselling and testing services", *J Acquir Immune Defic Syndr Hum Retrovirol,* 1998; 18(4): 384-8.

Elliott R. Trips and rights: *International human rights law, access to medicines, and the interpretation of the WTO agreement on trade-related aspects of intellectual property rights*, Montreal: Canadian HIV/AIDS Legal Network and AIDS Law Project (South Africa), 2001,

Family Health International et al., "What drives HIV in Asia? A summary of trends in sexual and drug-taking behaviours", Arlington: *Family Health International*, 2001.

FAO, *The impact of HIV/AIDS on food security*, 2001.

Fidler D.P., *International law and infectious diseases*, New York: Oxford University Press, 1999:210.

Fylkesnes, K., et al., "Declining HIV prevalence and risk behaviours in Zambia: evidence from surveillance and population-based surveys", *AIDS*; 15(7): 907–916, 2001.

Ghys P., et al., "HIV surveillance among female sex workers", *AIDS*; 15(3): 33–34, 2001.

Global Programme on AIDS. Consensus statement from the WHO/ UNICEF consultation on HIV transmission and breastfeeding. *Weekly Epidemiological Record,* 1992, 67:177–179.

Grosskurth H et al.. "Control of sexually transmitted diseases for HIV prevention: understanding the implications of the Mwanza and Rakai trials", *The Lancet,* 2000.

Gupta, Indrani. "Socio-economic impact of HIV/AIDS on Individuals: A Planning Perspective from India". In *The Looming Epidemic: the Impact of HIV and AIDS in India* (ed.), Peter Godwin, Mosaic, 1998.

Hecht R, Adeyi O., Semini I., "Making AIDS Part of the Global Development Agenda", *Finance & Development*; 39(1). Washington: IMF, 2002.

Hecht R., *Poverty, debt and AIDS—mainstreaming the epidemic and mobilising additional resources for the response*, Geneva, UNAIDS, Inter-Country Team for West and Central Africa, 2000.

Indian Council of Medical Research (ICMR), 1988, "Changing trends in sero-surveillance for HIV infection", *ICMR Bulletin* 18: 39.

Indrani, "The AIDS Epidemic and the Economic Burden of Treatment in India", Presented at the Meeting of the UNAIDS Reference Group on Economics, Cuernavaca, Mexico, February 2001.

International Council of AIDS Service Organisations (ICASO), *An advocate's guide to the international guidelines on HIV/AIDS and human rights*, Toronto: ICASO, 1999.

International Covenant on Economic, Social and Cultural Rights, adopted by General Assembly resolution 2200A (XXI) of 16 December.1966: Article 2(1).

Jain K., *Tribal sex seller women and HIV/AIDS infection in India. Xth International conference on AIDS*, Yokohama, Japan, 1994.

Jana S., Bandyopadhyay N., Mukherjee S., Dutta N., Basu I., Saha A., "SID/HIV intervention with sex workers in West Bengal, India", *AIDS* 1998.

Janssen, R.S., Satten, G.A., Stramer, S.L., Rawal, B.D., O'Brien, T.R., Weiblen, B.J., et al, "New testing strategy to detect early HIV-1 infection for use in incidence estimates and for clinical and prevention purposes", *JAMA* 1998; 280: 42-8.

Kirby J., "Human rights and the HIV paradox", *Lancet,* 1996.

Kumar M.S., Mudaliar, S., Thayagarajan, S.P., Kumar S., Selvanayagam A., "Rapid assessment and response to injecting drug use in Madras, South India", *International Journal of Drug Policy*, 11, 1–2: pp 83–98, 2002.

Loewenson R., Whiteside A. *HIV/AIDS. Implications for poverty reduction*, New York, UNDP, 2001.

Mann JM., Human rights and AIDS: the future of the pandemic. In: Mann J.M., Gruskin S., Grodin M.A., Annas G.J., *Health and human rights*, New York and London: Routledge, 1999:221.

MAP, *The status and trends of HIV/AIDS/STI epidemics in Asia and the Pacific*, October 4 2001, Melbourne, Australia.

Martinez, P.M., Torres, A.R., Oritz de Lejarazu. R., Montoya A., Martin, J.F., Eiros J.M., "Human immunodeficiency virus antibody testing by enzyme-linked fluorescent and Western blot assays using serum, gingival-crevicular transudate, and urine samples", *J Clin Microbiol*, 1999;37(4):1100-6.

Monitoring the AIDS Pandemic (MAP), "The Status and Trends of HIV/AIDS/STI Epidemics in Asia and the Pacific", Provisional Report. Melbourne, 2001.

National AIDS Control Organisation, *Combating HIV/AIDS in India, 2000–2001*, Ministry of Health and Family Welfare. National AIDS Control Organisation, Government of India.

National Committee for Clinical Laboratory Standards, "Procedures and devices for the collection of diagnostic blood specimens by skin puncture", *NCCLS document H4-A4*, 1999.

National Committee for Clinical Laboratory Standards, "Procedures for the handling and process of blood specimens; Approved guidelines", *NCCLS document*, H 18-A. 1990.

National Family Health Survey –2 (1998–1999), International Institute of Population Sciences. Mumbai.

Newell M.L., Rogers M. Pregnancy and HIV infection: a European consensus on management. *AIDS* 2002; 16:S1-S18.

Office of the United Nations Commissioner for Human Rights/ UNAIDS, "HIV/AIDS and Human Rights International Guidelines". Second International Consultation on HIV/AIDS and Human Rights, Geneva, 23–25 September. Geneva: United Nations, 1998.

Panda S., Bijaya L., Devi, N.S., et al., "Interface between drug use and sex work in Manipur, *National Medical Journal of India*. Vol 14: No 4, 2001.

Panda, S., etal., "HIV, hepatitis B and sexual practice in the street-recruited injecting drug users of Calcutta: risk perception versus observed risks", *International Journal STD & AIDS*. April. 9(4): 214–218, 1998.

Ramasundaram S., "Can India avoid being devastated by HIV", *British Medical Journal,* 324: 182–183 (26 January), 2002.

Reid G., Costigan G., *Revisiting 'The Hidden Epidemic': A Situation Assessment of Drug Use in Asia in the context of HIV/AIDS*, The Centre for Harm Reduction, The Burnet Institute, Australia, January 2002.

Respess, R.A., Rayfield, M.A., Dondero, T.J., "Laboratory testing and rapid HIV assays: applications for HIV surveillance in hard-to-reach populations", *AIDS* 2001; 15 (suppl 3):S49-S59.

Richmond J., and McKinney, R. , (ed.), *Biosafety in microbiological and biomedical laboratories*, Washington (DC):U.S. Government Printing Office; 1993.

Rose N.R., Conway de Macario E., Folds J.D., Lane H.C., Nakamura R.M.; editors. *Manual of clinical laboratory immunology*. 5th ed. Washington (DC): ASM Press; 1997.

Salama ,P., Dondero, T., "HIV surveillance in complex emergencies", *AIDS*; 15(3): S4–12.

Salunke, S.R., Shaukat M., Hira S.K., Jagtap, M.R., "HIV/AIDS in India: A country responds to a challenge", *AIDS*; 12 (Suppl B), 1998.

Second International Consultation on HIV/AIDS and Human Rights (Geneva, 23-25 September 1996). Report of the Secretary-General (E/CN.4/1997/37). Geneva: United Nations, 1997.

Stetler H.C., Granade T.C., Nunez C.A., Meza R, Terrell S., Amador L., et al. Field evaluation of rapid HIV serologic tests for screening and confirming HIV-1 infection in Honduras. *AIDS* 1997;11:369-75.

Suniti Solomon, et.al., "HIV in India", *Special Contribution*, Volume 10 Issue 3 July/August 2002.

Tam, M.R., "Serological and biomolecular detection of human immunodeficiency virus types 1 and 2", Seattle (WA): *Programme for Appropriate Technology in Health (PATH)*. June 1999.

Third International Conference on AIDS INDIA. Chennai. India, December 1–5, 2001.

Times of India, State orders HIV infection enquiry at blood banks, (Kolkata) 5 March, 2002.

UNAIDS, "Innovative approaches to HIV prevention", *Best Practice Collection*, Geneva, 2000.

UNAIDS, *A Multi-Ministerial Strategy to the Expanded Response to HIV/AIDS. HIV/AIDS Development in Asia and the Pacific: A lengthening shadow*, Geneva, 2001.

UNAIDS, *AIDS Epidemic Update 2001*, Geneva, 2001.

UNAIDS, *Children and young people in a world of AIDS*, Geneva, 2001.

UNAIDS, *HIV Testing Methods: UNAIDS Technical Update*, (UNAIDS Best Practice Collection Technical Update). Geneva: UNAIDS, November 1997.

UNAIDS, *The UNAIDS guide to the United Nations human rights machinery,* Geneva, 1997.

UNAIDS, UNICEF and WHO, *HIV and infant feeding. A policy statement developed collaboratively by UNAIDS, UNICEF and WHO*, Geneva, UNAIDS, 1997

UNAIDS, *United Nations-Facilitated Response to HIV/AIDS, STD and Drug Use in Central Asian Countries*, (Kazakhstan, Kyrgyzstan, Tajikistan, Turkmenistan and Uzbekistan), Geneva, 1999.

UNAIDS, *Workplan- 1999–2001. A Strategic Response to the HIV epidemic by the government of India, the UN and its development partners in India.*

UNAIDS/Inter-ParliamentaryUnion, 1999, *Handbook for legislators on HIV/AIDS, law and human rights: action to combat HIV/AIDS in view of its devastating human, economic and social impact*, Geneva, 2001.

UNAIDS/WHO (2001), *Sources and prices of selected drugs and diagnostics for people living with HIV/AIDS*, Geneva: UNAIDS (UNAIDS/01.65E).

UNAIDS/WHO , *Guidelines for second generation HIV surveillance*, Geneva: UNAIDS/WHO. WHO/ CDS/CSR/EDC/2000.

UNAIDS/WHO, *AIDS Epidemic Update*, December 2001.

UNDP, "HIV/AIDS: *Implications for Poverty Reduction*, New York, 2001.

UNDP, Human Development Report, 2001. New York, 2001.

UNICEF, *The epidemiology of HIV at the start of the 21st century*, New York, 2002.

UNICEF/UNAIDS, *South Asia: The HIV/AIDS Epidemic*, 2001.

United Nations General Assembly, *Declaration of Commitment on HIV/AIDS: 'Global Crisis—Global Action*, 2001.

United Nations General Assembly, *Declaration of commitment on HIV/AIDS*, New York: United Nations, 2001: paragraphs 16, 58 (A/RES/S-26/2).

United Nations High Commissioner for Human Rights. *The protection of human rights in the context of human immunodeficiency virus*

(HIV) and acquired immunodeficiency syndrome (AIDS). Commission on Human Rights resolution 1997/33. Geneva: Office of the United Nations High Commissioner for Human Rights, 1997 (E/CN.4/RES/1997/33).

Universal Declaration of Human Rights, adopted and proclaimed by the United Nations General Assembly Resolution 217 A (III) of 10 December 1948.

USAID, "Efforts to Address the Needs of Children Affected by HIV/AIDS", Washington: The Synergy Project, 2001.

Webb D., Elliott L., *Learning to Live: Monitoring and evaluating HIV/AIDS programmes for young people*, London: Save the Children/Department for International Development/UNAIDS, 2000.

WHO, *Antiretroviral drugs and the prevention of mother-to-child transmission of HIV infection in resource-constrained settings*, 7 January 2004.

WHO, *Biosafety guidelines for diagnostic and research laboratories working with HIV*, Geneva: 1991. *WHO AIDS Series* 9.

WHO/GPA., *Statement from the consultation on testing and counselling for HIV infection*, Geneva 16-18 November 1992.

WHO/UNAIDS, *Prevention of Mother-to-Child Transmission of HIV: Selection and Use of Nevirapine*, Geneva, 2001.

World Bank, *Confronting AIDS: public priorities in a global epidemic*, Oxford: Oxford University Press for the World Bank, 1999.

World Bank, *Confronting AIDS. Public Priorities in a Global Epidemic*, 1997.

World Bank, *World Development Report 2000/2001: Attacking poverty*, Washington, 2001.

World Health Organisation and Joint United Nations Programme on HIV/AIDS, *Guidelines for Using HIV Testing Technologies in Surveillance: Selection, Evaluation, and Implementation*, 2001.

Index